NURSE'S ORDER

THE ULTIMATE EXPERT GUIDE TO HEALTH.

Michael Huxley, BA, BSc, RNA

Copyright 2012 by Michael Huxley

Contents.

Part 4 - So what now?

Introduction.

Living a healthy lifestyle, eating a good, healthy diet, getting enough exercise and being fit and strong. They sound like such simple concepts, don't they? We all know that is what we should be doing, yet so many of us fail to do so for so many reasons. I imagine if you are reading this book then you want to tone up or get fit? Maybe you want to lose a little weight or simply become a little bit healthier but you don't really know how to go about it properly? Well don't worry that is what this book is here for, to give you the no nonsense truth on diet, exercise and health, to separate the fact from the fad, and to give you the basic facts and real information you will need to transform your body, eating habits, exercise routine and your life. It isn't here to confuse you with technical jargon or medical terminology because I believe that the knowledge needed to live a healthy lifestyle does not have to be difficult or confusing, but it will not pander to the myths and half truths out there and will not accept excuses or fads. The advice contained in this book is simple common sense advice backed up by clinical knowledge and evidence that all of you, regardless of your fitness levels or health at the moment, can use to improve your quality of life.

I constantly get asked how to exercise, what constitutes a healthy diet, how to lose weight and a whole variety of questions in between. The reasons people ask me vary almost as much as the questions themselves, some need the advice to counteract a health problem, others just want to get a little bit healthier, and some just want to lose weight and look good. Every single person will have a unique motivation for wanting to adopt a healthier lifestyle and there is nothing wrong with any of these reasons. It doesn't matter why you choose to do so, only that you put in the commitment to make that change. All it takes is time, a bit of effort on your part and a bit of knowledge. There are no quick fixes, no short cuts, no one day diets or fads that will shed the flab and give you a perfect body overnight. But with the right information and the right tools, you can reach your ideal weight, get that perfect beach body, fit into that dress or be as strong or as fit as you want to be, and more importantly you can live a healthy lifestyle and save yourself a multitude of health problems down the road.

You have already taken that important first step by arming yourself with the right knowledge about a healthy diet, exercise and living a complete, balanced healthy lifestyle. All you need now is the self determination and the will to put it into practice, because this book can't do everything for you. Only you can do that. No one has a little bloke in a Staff Sergeant uniform following them round, bellowing 'get away from that fridge!' 'Put that cupcake down lardy!' 'Go for a run! Move, move, move!' Or if they do they are keeping it a huge secret from the rest of us. Only you can make these changes, only you can eat a healthy, balanced diet and join that gym or go for a run. Only you can have the willpower to make yourself thinner, stronger, fitter and healthier, but I will guarantee that if you do, if you follow the advice in this book, keep it up over the long term and incorporate these factors into a long term healthy lifestyle, then you will be much happier, much healthier, and less likely to need my professional services in the future!

That's right, apart from healthy living and exercise being a big part of my own personal life, I'm also a qualified and registered nurse, so health and wellbeing are a big part of my professional life too. Poor lifestyle choices such as poor diet, smoking, drinking to excess, obesity, sedentary lifestyles and lack of exercise have a profound impact on people's health, and one of the biggest challenges we face as health professionals is combating the illnesses and long term health complications of those who make poor lifestyle choices throughout their life.

It is no secret that the nation as a whole is hardly a healthy one. A general lack of physical activity, unhealthy, unbalanced diets and unhealthy lifestyle habits such as smoking and drinking to excess all contribute to Britain being an unhealthy nation. As a registered nurse I see all too often the direct effects of these poor lifestyles on people's health, and have seen how they have contributed to numerous conditions such as metabolic disorder, obesity, COPD, diabetes, heart disease and many more. What annoys me is the knowledge that many of these conditions can be severely reduced or even halted altogether with the simple introduction of a healthy lifestyle. I cannot stress enough how easily it is to link the causes of so many conditions and illnesses somewhere along the line to poor lifestyle choices.

As a registered nurse I constantly get family members, friends and acquaintances coming up to me and asking for advice on a condition they have, especially when I'm not in work and all I want to do is remind people it's my day off. Often they tell me intimate things I really don't wish to know about or shove a hideous carbuncle in my face and asking what I think. Not ideal if you want to relax or are about to tuck into a nice meal! I feel sometimes like the TV doctor who looks at embarrassing bodies, except I don't get the fame or a nice wad of cash from the TV companies. Not that I mind really, at least I'm helping. That's what I keep telling myself anyway as I bang my head against a brick wall in full knowledge that most people won't even follow the advice I give them.

That's because a large part of this advice is often devoted to diet, exercise and healthy living. Even if the question is about a particular condition, it will often come back down to lifestyle and health at some point. And yes, I freely admit I get frustrated when I have to fight through a brick wall of myths and half-truths from the sea of fad diets, self help books and celebrity DVDs that are out there, especially when I know those very same people who asked my advice will often nod politely and then completely ignore it because it will involve effort or change on their part.

Incorporating a healthy diet and exercise into your daily routine will most probably involve at least some effort on your part, but the real secret is that this change is actually not that hard once you start, and once you do you will find that living a healthy lifestyle is easy! Incorporating little things at first will soon become normal to you, and then you just build on that. Eating a healthy diet and getting to a healthy weight is quite simple, it will just take a bit of willpower and time, and exercise is absolutely nothing to worry about. Some of you might even enjoy it!

This is what this book is about, this is what I aim to tell you. This isn't just a normal diet book, this isn't just an exercise manual, this is a book on how to completely overhaul yourself to live a good, balanced, healthy lifestyle. The message is simple, eat a healthy balanced diet, exercise, and get a good work/life balance, and you will be much fitter, much healthier, and much happier. This is not breaking news, this is not some great new discovery that has just been made. This is simple common knowledge, and I would argue even basic common sense. People know this, yet the advice often gets ignored, or confused with a maze of myths and half truths.

In the pages that follow, I will give you the information you need to make all of these changes in the right way. I will help you find that perfect balanced diet and give you the information you need to make informed choices about what and when you eat. I will help you shed those pounds and improve your fitness levels. I will give you the information you need to become much healthier, and along the way I hope I can shed some light on some common diet and fitness myths and hopefully stop you from seeing me and my colleagues in a professional capacity at some point in the future.

Part 1 - Understanding your body and your health.

How many of us truly know our own body? And I mean really know it? I'm not talking about the delusional ideal that you imagine when you suck in your gut in front of the mirror or convince yourself that it is the label on those Jeans that are wrong because you should be able to fit into them! I'm talking about truly understanding your body and how it works. I'm talking about understanding what your natural body shape is and what your body fat levels are and should be. I'm talking about having an awareness of how healthy your cardiovascular, metabolic, muscular and skeletal systems are, and knowing how all those essential internal functions that your body performs are working optimally.

Having a basic understanding of your own body and the factors that make up how fit and healthy you are or even what makes you unhealthy or ill, is extremely important in maintaining a healthy lifestyle, and one that is often seriously overlooked in favour of the fad diet of the week. Without this basic knowledge, you will not be able to implement the right tools, or avoid all the myths, lies and misinformation out there, in order for you to become fit and healthy and truly transform your quality of life.

How many of you, and be honest with yourself here, have picked up one of those nonsense magazines and read about the amazing new wonder diet that some non entity celeb swears by (and then uses airbrushed photos to convince you it works)? How many of you read it and thought that is a great idea, I'll try that? How many of you have starved yourself in the mistaken belief that you would lose weight, or actually started exercising but quit after a session or two because it wasn't working and you didn't understand why? How many of you have suffered, or are suffering from an illness or condition such as diabetes, COPD, heart disease or any number of conditions, and then wondered why you got it, completely ignoring the fact that you are severely overweight, smoke 50 a day, have a poor diet or never exercise? How many? I'll bet it is a lot.

This is why to understand how to live a healthy lifestyle, eat a healthy diet and exercise well, you have to understand the basics of why it is necessary to do so. It is important to understand what your body is, what it does, and how it is affected by positive or negative lifestyle choices.

This book isn't intended to guide you through the knowledge it would take to earn a degree in medicine or nursing. That information is certainly out there if you wish to compound this basic knowledge with a more in depth understanding of anatomy and health, but in this book I just want to give you a basic understanding of what it is to be healthy. I especially want to dispel the myths and half truths used to fuel the fad diet industry in various magazines and DVDs.

The first thing to understand is how simple and interconnected a lot of things are. So many health problems, illnesses, injuries and diseases are all fundamentally affected at some point by basic health, diet and fitness. Poor lifestyle choices lead to being unfit, overweight or obese, that leads to a variety of long term health conditions and they in turn lead to more serious health problems. So let's get right back down to the basics.

Body shape.

The concept of body shape is one that is familiar to most of us, but just as confusing in equal measure. We are constantly bombarded with a variety of body shapes and types in the mass media, and not always in a positive way either. We have all seen the images of ultra skinny models or muscular, six pack toting men. You may have been told that you have an hourglass figure, a vase figure, a 'V' shape or a fuller figure (although even I wouldn't dare say that to a woman, I value my nose too much!) I've even heard of skittle and lollipop shaped figures! You may have heard about special wonder diets based on certain body shapes named after fruits, you may think you have an 'apple', a 'pear' or a 'banana' body. Okay I don't know where the last one came from but the fact remains that there is a lot of confusion out there, with very little understanding of the true facts.

The simple fact is that regardless of all the nonsense names and labels that have been applied to them by fad diets and fashion programmes over the years, there are only three basic categories of body shapes, known as somatotypes, with slight differences for each gender. The three extremes of somatotypes or body shapes are Ectomorph, Mesomorph and Endomorph.

Male Ectomorphs: Usually skinny and lean, with very little natural body fat and thin limbs. Ectomorphs find it very difficult to gain and maintain large muscle mass, and will usually gain and hold fat around their stomachs and waist. Ectomorphs have high endurance levels and are often faster than other body types.

Female Ectomorph: Slim frame and petite, with thin limbs and hips and small, if any, curves. Any excess body fat is usually held around the stomach. Often have greater levels of endurance and stamina. Imagine long distance runners for example, that ultra lean build and lack of body fat is a typical example of an Ectomorph.

Male Mesomorph: Naturally muscular and athletic with large frames, often have barrel chests and thick, muscular limbs. Mesomorphs find it easy to gain large muscle mass quickly, but also gain body fat very easily too unless regular training occurs. Can easily adapt to most fitness regimes.

Female Mesomorph: Naturally curvy with wide hips and chest, but a slimmer stomach. This is the classic hourglass shape that certain fad diets tend to promote. Like their male counterparts, female Mesomorphs can also gain body fat very easily.

Male Endomorph: Usually short, but not always, Endomorphs are typically round in shape and often have a naturally higher percentage of body fat. Endomorphs often find it very difficult to lose weight.

Female Endomorph: Again usually short, with a round, curvaceous figure. What certain magazines usually call the apple shape. Female endomorphs tend to have larger chests and stomachs, but narrow hips. Tend to gain weight on the chest or bottom, and find it easy to put weight on, but difficult to lose it.

These are the true categories of actual body types, and are the extremes of each example. Many people don't conform to the total extreme of one category or another, but fall somewhere in between along a sliding scale. For example, you can get someone who is balanced somewhere between being a lean Ectomorph and a muscular Mesomorph.

These somatotypes become relatively important when determining your own fitness regime, for example you may need more cardiovascular workouts if you are an Ectomorph, to counteract the body fat gain that is very easy for that body shape, but it is even more important when determining your fitness goals and having a realistic idea of what your body can look like at its best, or just as importantly, what it won't look like.

There is a great deal of confusion about how to achieve that 'perfect' body, especially since not many people can even define what a perfect body is! I've lost count of the amount of times I have met guys in the gym who want to build huge muscles to look like a bodybuilder or women who want to starve themselves to look like a supermodel or one of those ridiculously ill looking size zero celebs! That is a craze I have never, and will never understand.

The problem is, that supposed 'ideal' body shape will never happen for many people. There is no point trying to get a body like that celebrity you saw in that film or that ultra skinny model who swears she 'eats like a horse', because you may not have the right body shape. It is completely unrealistic for some people to want to be ultra skinny, or have huge breasts, or massive muscles, it just won't happen. Not without a significant amount of unnatural, assisted help. A male Ectomorph will never have muscles like Schwarzenegger for example, and a female Mesomorph will never look like Kate Moss, not without starving herself and becoming extremely ill, anyway. The best thing you can do is learn about your own body type, your own individual shape, and mould that to be the best it possibly can be. It doesn't matter if you don't look like someone else, because you will know you have made the best out of what your own individual body shape is. Great, now I sound like I'm on an American daytime chat show.

The specific body type you are as well as your specific shape and measurements involve more than just how you want to look. They can have a very real impact on your health too. Studies have shown that where you carry your fat is just as important for health implications as how much of it you are carrying. Those who tend to hold fat around their stomach for example tend to be at greater risk of health problems such as Diabetes, Cardiovascular disease and so on.

The concept of fat, and being fat, is often just as confusing to people as body shape. Sure, we all get the basic concept, we all know that the chunk who took up two seats when sitting next to us on the plane home from our holiday is fat, but when it comes down to it there are a lot of myths and half truths out there that can be extremely confusing.

Many people who pick up a book like this, or nervously go down to the gym for the first time or start that fad diet, do so because they want to lose weight. We have all at some point looked at ourselves and wished we were a little thinner, or know we are overweight but don't have the knowledge, tools, or more importantly the willpower to do anything about it. Obesity is a huge problem in society now, and for many long term health conditions this is where things start to go wrong. Of course, diet and exercise play a part in controlling this, but let's first understand exactly what we mean when we talk about being fat or overweight.

So am I fat? What exactly is overweight?

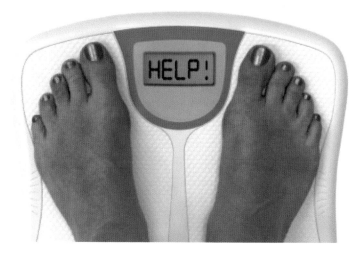

There is a lot of misunderstanding about fat out there. People often get confused about exactly what constitutes being fat or overweight and if their individual weight means they are actually fat or not. To be honest I'm not surprised. There is so much misinformation going around, so many myths and half truths, some of them even peddled by the health industry itself, that quite frankly it would take a minor miracle not to be confused by it all. To understand the difference between weight and fat, and exactly what constitutes being overweight, we again have to go right back to the basics.

Fat is essentially adipose tissue, that is all. There are a variety of types, all having different uses, but don't worry you don't need a degree in physiology to understand it. The three basic types you need to concern yourself with are intramuscular fat, which lays in between your muscles, visceral fat around our internal organs (and our stomach), and subcutaneous fat which is just under the skin. It is these last two that most people tend to be concerned about, whether they know it or not. When you look in the mirror and see those tyre like bulges popping out of your dress or that huge thing blocking the mirror out that you swear isn't your own backside, that's good old subcutaneous fat. When you notice that gut hanging over your belt on the other hand, that is visceral or abdominal fat, and it is these which you have to maintain at a healthy level.

The reason men and women tend to differ in where they put fat on (and also struggle to get it off) is predominantly down to hormone differences between the two genders. Unfortunately ladies you naturally have more fat than guys do. Don't shoot the messenger, I'm not calling you fat! That's all down to physiology (and your hormones). Sorry about that. But don't worry too much about that, you need to understand that it isn't about having fat or not, it is about having the right amount of fat that is right for you and your individual body.

> Top tip: Throw away the scales! Yes you heard me, just throw them out of the window (making sure you don't hit next doors cat in the process!) Weight in and of itself is not important at all when determining how fat, thin or healthy you are. Your total weight is made up of much more than just fat and includes muscle and fluid too, and muscle is much denser than fat.

Basically, there are many different types of fat and you have to keep in mind that some of it at certain levels is actually quite good for you, so starving yourself to a size zero isn't the best idea either. So what exactly is a healthy amount of fat I hear you all cry? What is the ideal amount of body fat so we can have that lean, toned body but still be healthy?

The Body Mass Index (BMI).

The method of measuring weight that the vast majority of people will be familiar with is the BMI, or the Body Mass Index. This basically involves weighing yourself and then comparing your weight against your height. This method is extremely common, and will be seen in any weight loss club, many gyms, and surprisingly even GP surgeries and hospitals. However, this method is extremely dated and somewhat inaccurate. The statistics used for the current BMI were based on a very small population study over 40 years ago and doesn't take into account many individual differences such as the distribution between lean mass and adipose tissue, somatotype (body type) or muscle mass, and although muscle weighs the same as fat, it is much denser so it takes a smaller amount of muscle to weigh as much as a larger amount of fat. This is the reason some people find when they start exercising and losing fat, they actually gain a little weight or at least don't lose any because of the muscle they have toned and built up through exercising. According to the BMI chart for example, almost every professional Rugby player is clinically obese! I'm certainly not going to be the one who tells them that! But don't worry, as you exercise, build muscle and lose body fat, you may still weigh the same or perhaps even more, but you will still find those inches coming off your waist or that you can actually fit into those jeans without the aid of a team of people pulling and squeezing you into them.

The BMI isn't perfect, but it can still be used as a rough guess for the average person. I would not recommend using it as the sole basis for determining if you are overweight or not however, as your weight isn't just about how fat or thin you are. I would recommend that it should only ever be used as a rough guide to then compare to much more accurate and comprehensive data. This is where specific body fat levels come into play.

Body fat levels.

There are a number of different ways to specifically measure body fat as opposed to weight, but the most common are skin fold callipers (the old pinch an inch tool) through to bioelectric impedance analysis (BIA) tools, which use electrical flow impedance to see exactly how much of your body is actually made up of fat (muscle has a higher conductivity to fat, so muscle is not counted as it is with measuring weight alone). You can get hold of these machines quite easily yourself, or if you don't want to buy one, a lot of modern gyms should have them. A few GP surgeries or walk in clinics may have them too although not all do. Basically once you have measured the amount of fat you actually have, this is then converted into a percentage and is measured against a chart such as this.

Body fat chart (Adults)

Essential Fat Level Women - 10 - 13%

Essential Fat Level Men - 2 - 5%

Athlete Level Women - 14 - 20%

Athlete Level Men - 6 - 13%

Fit Level Women - 21 - 24%

Fit Level Men - 14 - 17%

Average Level Women - 25 - 31%

Average Level Men - 18 - 24%

Obese   Level Women - 32% plus.

Obese Level Men - 25% plus.

Basically, anything below 10 - 13% body fat in women and 2 - 5% in men is considered 'underfat' or unhealthy, and anything above 31% in women and 24 % in men is considered obese. So just as much as someone who is obese is considered unhealthy and needs to lose some body fat, the exact same is true for those who have far too little and need to put some 'weight' on. Just look at the ultra skinny celebs you see in magazines or some of the guys you see every single spring who walk around with their tops off the second the sun comes out, thinking they look like Gods' gift because they have a six pack. Here's a big neon message to all of you, you don't look like an underwear model, you are not sexy, more often than not you look ill. Go and get a good healthy meal down you. The ideal body fat level in adults is obviously to be within those two extremes. Exactly where you fall on the chart will obviously depend on how much physical activity you do and on your diet, but as usual the middle ground of 'fit' is arguably the best, unless you are a professional athlete of course (in which case, why are you reading this? Get back to your training!)

As long as you are within a healthy body fat range, then don't worry too much if you don't look like that skinny celeb off the TV, or you can't get into that ridiculous size zero dress. It doesn't matter. People are very individual and unique, with a wide range of heights and body shapes, so not everyone can. Like I said earlier, this is all down to body shape too. Having a healthy range of body fat, regardless of what height, weight or body shape you are means that you have the exact amount of fat you need to maintain a healthy lifestyle for you as an individual. Not too much, but not too little either. This is what it really means to be healthy and comfortable within your own individual body, not the American habit that many obese people adopt of saying 'I'm comfortable in my own body', usually said with a self delusional head wobble as an excuse not to do anything about being too fat.

Waist to hip ratio.

Now that you have a basic understanding of what fat is, how to measure it, and how much fat you should have to be considered healthy, just to make things a little more confusing, you also need to consider where on your body fat is stored too. Current research and guidelines state that it isn't just the amount of fat that you have, it is where you carry it that counts too. This is because fat that is carried around the waist, visceral or abdominal fat, is an indicator of the level of fat that is being carried around your vital organs. So as well as body shape and body fat levels, the waist to hip ratio is also important for determining health. This means measuring your hips and measuring your waist, and then being completely honest with the results. No pretending that 38 inches really looks like 34! As a rough indicator just on waist size alone, the ideal waist measurement for men is less than 37 inches, 37 - 40 inches is considered high, and above 40 inches or more is considered too high, or obese. In women, less than 32 inches is ideal, 32 - 35 inches is high, and above 35 inches is too high or obese.

Again, these measurements are different for men and women, but to get a slightly more accurate figure what you need to do next is get a tape measure and hold it around your true waist (about where your belly button is) and mark that number down, and then do the same for your hips and divide the waist number by the hip number. This is your waist to hip ratio.

Once you have divided this waist measurement by your hip measurement, then you should end up with a specific number.

For example, a female waist measurement of 33 inches divided by a hip measurement of 38 inches equals 0.87. If you are male and that number is 1.0 or above, then you are carrying too much fat around your middle, if you are female and the number is 0.85 or more, it means you are carrying too much fat around your middle too.

I know this variety of ways and tools for measuring your body fat levels and determining how healthy or relatively fat you are can be confusing, but it does get simple once you get used to it. In an average person, a healthy level of body fat should pretty much correlate with a healthy hip to waist ratio and the BMI anyway, but the most important point to remember is that as long as your body fat levels are somewhere within the athlete or fit category, then great, if they are average but your waist/hip ratio is okay and you are otherwise healthy, then that is great too. If they are not, then you will need to adjust your diet accordingly and get some exercise. It is all about understanding your own individual body, using different measuring tools to get a better idea of what your current state of health or fat levels are, and understanding what is, and what isn't healthy for you as an individual.

But I'm fat and I'm fit?

This is an issue where a lot of people understandably get confused. Especially with the media occasionally having a frenzy of sensationalist headlines that really do nothing but misinform people. There are certainly Sumo wrestlers in Japan who are fitter than a lot of people half their size, and likewise there are thin people who would collapse in a fit of wheezing after running round the block and have numerous health problems to boot. Whilst it is absolutely true that moderate levels of exercise at least can greatly reduce or even halt disease or mortality risks, any excess weight will still have an effect on diseases like diabetes and cardiovascular diseases such as COPD. So what is going on? What it boils down to is that as important as body fat levels are in maintaining a healthy lifestyle, there is more to being fit and healthy than being fat or skinny.

Cardiovascular fitness, which is something I'll come to in a later chapter, is essential. It is certainly possible for a person with a moderate to high level of body fat levels to have a higher level of cardiovascular fitness than someone who is slim. Without getting too technical, if you are overweight, but you have better endurance, lung capacity, VO2 max and a higher lactate threshold than someone with less body fat levels than you, you would still technically be fitter than them with a higher level of cardiovascular fitness. However, you have to remember that the excess body fat will still cause you problems such as arthritis from the impact training of running and other chronic disease, and you would be even fitter still if you lost the extra body fat.

The biggest cause of confusion in all of this is metabolic health. more so than cardiovascular fitness, it is this more

24

than anything which indicates if you are healthy or not regardless of whether you are fat or thin. This means that you should have normal blood pressure, normal triglyceride levels, low cholesterol levels and normal levels of blood sugar, and do not display the same risks of developing heart disease, cancer, cardiovascular illness, diabetes and high blood pressure that most people who are considered overweight or obese do. This isn't to say that you still shouldn't try and maintain a healthy body fat percentage because having too much still raises your chances of getting all these conditions and more, but it does mean that fat, or 'weight' isn't the only consideration when it comes to overall health.

So what is metabolic health?

Metabolic health doesn't refer to your actual metabolism, they are two different things. Metabolic health refers to the condition of the inner workings of your body, such as cholesterol, blood pressure, blood sugar and other factors that you need to keep healthy so that your body runs at its best and you don't develop numerous long term conditions. Metabolic homeostasis is all about how your bodily systems function and regulate themselves. It really isn't all that complicated, but it has led to so many health myths and misunderstandings.

Poor metabolic health leads to a variety of illnesses and long term health conditions, and the various components that make up your metabolic health as a whole are almost always affected by lifestyle choices such as diet and exercise, smoking, drinking to excess, drug taking and obesity. But the simple truth is, by living a healthy lifestyle, eating a well balanced diet and exercising, you can take control of all of these things and ensure your body is healthy and fit. To do this however, you also need a basic understanding of each of the components that make up your metabolic health, how they can make you healthy or unhealthy, and what you can do to keep them running at their best.

Blood pressure.

Blood pressure is something that most people will be familiar with at some point or another. Many of you may have had it taken by a practice nurse or your GP, and many more will have seen it done on the TV, often wrongly, but at least you should be aware of what it is.

To explain these things in a little more detail, blood pressure is what health professionals consider as one of the basic vital signs and refers to the level of pressure that is available in your arteries to pump the blood around your body. An average adults normal blood pressure is considered between 110 - 140 systolic (the pressure when your heart beats and pumps your blood), and 70 - 85 diastolic (the level of pressure when your heart rests in between beats). You may hear this referred to as 120 over 80 for example if you have your blood pressure taken. However this is only a rough average and there is a 'buffer zone' around that average that is considered normal and healthy. Generally speaking, and without taking any other factors into account, a persistent level of 140/90 or more is considered high. Individual blood pressure is dependent on a variety of factors including clinical history, age and weight and is very individual to each person. Blood pressure can even vary during the day and will be affected by smoking, medication, stress and many other factors. It is not uncommon to have a patient have high blood pressure readings, just from the stress of having their blood pressure taken! This is why it is important not just to take it once, but to take it regularly over a period of time and gain a picture, or a pattern, of blood pressure readings.

High blood pressure, or hypertension, is one of the leading causes of heart disease, heart attacks and stroke. There are a variety of causes, including some genetic factors, but primarily almost always comes down to poor lifestyle choices. Obesity and being overweight, a poor diet, too much salt or alcohol and a lack of physical activity all contribute toward high blood pressure and is very serious as many people can live a normal life for many years without realising they have it. That is why it is important to live a healthy lifestyle and get your blood pressure checked regularly.

Cholesterol.

Cholesterol again is a leading cause of heart disease, heart attacks, stroke and other conditions. It is basically a fatty substance that is made in the body and carried around the bloodstream by proteins, which when combined make up one of two different lipoproteins, low density lipoproteins which are the harmful type of cholesterol, and high density lipoprotein which is the protective type. It is having too much of this low density lipoprotein (LDL) cholesterol which causes you harm and raises your risk of cardiovascular disease.

Without any other underlying medical conditions, high LDL cholesterol is caused predominantly by eating too much saturated fat in your diet. It really is as simple as that. By cutting down on saturated fat in your diet, eating oily fish and fibre, maintaining healthy body fat levels and getting regular exercise, you can reduce and maintain a healthy cholesterol level.

Blood sugar.

Your blood sugar levels, like blood pressure and cholesterol, are an integral part of your bodies system. Basically it refers to the amount of glucose in your blood, the primary source of energy for your body.

It is perfectly normal for blood sugar levels to fluctuate during the day, before and after mealtimes for example, and are the reason why you may feel tired in the morning or if you skipped lunch because your boss made you finish that work you just had to do. Maintaining these blood sugar levels by eating a healthy diet regularly throughout the day and getting regular exercise is important, especially vital if you already have Diabetes Mellitus.

High blood sugar, or hyperglycaemia, happens when there is too much glucose in the bloodstream. When diabetes is not an issue, the body is generally quite good at regulating blood sugar levels and will not be a problem in short, temporary bursts, if you have one too many fizzy drinks for example. However, if it persists over a long period of time then a wide variety of problems can occur, such as kidney and cardiovascular damage.

Low blood sugar, or hypoglycaemia, happens when there is too little glucose in the blood stream, and when medication or other medical conditions are not involved it is most often caused by skipping meals or fasting. That is why those ridiculous fad diets that involve not eating are so dangerous. Like hyperglycaemia, low blood sugar levels are most common in diabetics, but can occur in non diabetics too. Common symptoms generally involve tiredness or lethargy, but if it persists, can lead to confusion, dizziness, headaches and a variety of other symptoms of varying severity dependent on the individual.

When diabetes is a factor maintaining blood sugar levels becomes vital. Type 1 diabetes is where blood sugar cannot be controlled because the body cannot produce enough insulin and needs to be controlled via the injection of insulin. Type 2 diabetes is where the body cannot use the insulin that is produced. This type is far more common, and can be insulin, tablet or diet controlled. Type 3, or gestational diabetes occurs during pregnancy and is often transient and relatively uncommon.

Type 2 diabetes.

Type 1 diabetes which is genetic, and type 3, with its own set of obvious contributing factors are pretty much out of peoples control on whether they have it or not. Type 2 diabetes however, although some genetic factors do play a small part, is predominantly caused by poor lifestyle choices such as poor diet, lack of exercise and obesity. This is the type of diabetes that you run the risk of developing if you live a poor lifestyle, do not manage your blood sugar levels, eat a poor diet rich in sugary food and drink, and are obese over a long period of time.

Current research suggests that over the next ten years, type 2 diabetes will be an even larger health problem for the nation than it is now, as increasing numbers of younger people present themselves to their GP or practice nurse with the condition due primarily to poor lifestyle choices.

For many people who develop type 2 diabetes, it can be controlled through eating a healthy diet and exercising, this is commonly referred to as diet controlled diabetes. It is also important to note that before patients get to this stage, a healthy lifestyle may reverse the chances of developing it altogether. For other people however, medication will be required either in tablet or insulin injection form. Regardless of which type of diabetes you develop, a lifestyle change is essential. Regular exercise, maintaining healthy body fat levels, managing your blood sugar levels and eating a healthy, well balanced diet and managing carbohydrate intake are all essential.

If diabetes is not managed correctly through medication, a healthy lifestyle or both, the health risks that occur as a result can be severe, especially if left untreated over a long period of time.

Not controlling your blood sugar levels over a long period of time can affect the lining of the arteries, making them much more prone to becoming blocked. This is compounded by a poor diet, especially one high in cholesterol, and is a significant risk factor in stroke, myocardial infarction or heart attacks and cardiovascular disease.

Diabetic retinopathy and neuropathy are also significant health risks of having uncontrolled diabetes. Retinopathy can occur when the small blood vessels are damaged which in turn can damage the retina, even causing blindness in extreme cases. Seeing an Optician regularly is absolutely essential if you are diagnosed with diabetes. Neuropathy happens on a similar principle, where diabetes damages the nerves and vessels but this time the ones leading from your brain to your body. Basically this means the brain finds it harder to tell your body how to work, causing numbness or tingling, weakened muscles, a weak bladder and even impotence in men. In extreme cases, this nerve damage to the extremities can even lead to amputation of the limb, specifically the feet.

Nephropathy, or kidney disease is a serious complication of long term mismanaged diabetes or blood sugar levels. According to the World Health Organisation, diabetes is a leading cause of Kidney failure, with 10 - 20% of diabetics dying from this complication every year.

Living a healthy lifestyle, eating a healthy balanced diet and regular exercise is the key to managing diabetes, regardless of type. But it is much more than that, a healthy lifestyle is the key to maintaining whole metabolic health. It is the key to everything, from maintaining healthy bodily systems and preventing illness and disease, to controlling or even reversing various health conditions if they occur.

Metabolic health is just as important a consideration when you are determining your overall health. Yes 'weight' and body fat levels are essential, but it is important to remember that it is not the only thing that you need to consider. It is all about developing a full picture of your whole health.

So what exactly is my metabolism, and why is it making me fat?

You may have heard many myths about your metabolism, as well as many excuses. 'It's not my fault I'm fat, I have a slow metabolism!' Or 'You are so lucky you have a good metabolism that makes you thinner!' It's rubbish. Nonsense. A complete fallacy. A lie that fat people tell themselves to give them an excuse not to do anything about being fat. A little harsh? Probably. But the truth is people need to stop making excuses. They need to look at some real home truths and take an honest look at themselves and their weight. Excuses will not cut it anymore, not if you want to lose weight and become healthier.

A big part of this is to stop using your metabolism as an excuse, and take the time to understand its important role in burning up the calories you consume during the day.

> Myth buster! It is a complete fallacy that overweight people have a slow metabolism and thin people have a fast metabolism. In fact, studies have shown that both lean and fat people have similar metabolic rates.

Your metabolism is just your bodies way of using up the calories you consume during the day so that your heart can keep beating, your lungs can keep pumping oxygen in and out of you and you can run about and do all the little things you do during your day (not including physical activity, which is a separate type of energy). Simple really, isn't it?

You may have heard of the term 'metabolic rate'. Well it's pretty much the same thing. It just refers to the specific rate in which your metabolism uses up your consumed calories. If you consume more calories than your body needs in any given day, then your metabolism will simply take what it needs, and then the rest will be stored as fat for use at a later date.

> Myth buster! Special diets, supplements or pills can increase metabolism, can't they? No, they absolutely can't. And many of them may even have unwanted negative side effects.

The only real way to improve your metabolism, and therefore the rate in which your body burns up calories, is by becoming fitter and stronger. Basically, the fitter and stronger you are, the more efficient your body is in keeping you at a healthy weight, fit and healthy. Sorry, I know that seems backward and really unfair, but I did warn you there were no quick fixes. Basically by increasing muscle mass in contrast to body fat levels, (also known as body composition), you will increase your basal metabolic rate and will burn up calories more efficiently.

Part 2 - Diet.

Diet. It's a scary word. The term itself conjures up nightmares of endlessly counting calories or starving yourself. It makes you think of those ridiculous magazine articles and celebrity fad diets which encourage you to make yourself ill eating nothing but cabbage or cutting out carbs completely. You will have no doubt seen a thousand and one variations on this theme, diets promising that perfect beach body or making you look ten years younger if you stick to their version of the latest fad. Many of you may have tried one of these fad diets, then probably broke down in tears because you crack after a day or two when you realise it isn't working and you feel rubbish, and then reach for that cake, not a slice, the whole cake!

It really does not have to be like that. The term 'diet' is just that, it is just a term used to describe what we eat and drink on a daily basis. It is not a specific way of eating or a period of time eating a specific type of food. So I'm going to let you in on a little badly kept health secret that no one in the 'diet' industry will want you to know. You don't need to follow a plan. You don't need to eat only 'specially prepared' pre packaged meals or pay out vast amounts of money each week to get weighed and get a round of applause from a load of people you don't know, unless you really enjoy that sort of thing. You don't even need to deny yourself certain foods! Instead of looking at the term 'diet' in fear and automatically assuming you have to starve yourself, why not build up an idea of what a healthy diet consists of, and then eat reasonable portions dependent on your own individual needs? This advice is equally applicable to those with special dietary requirements for religious or ethical reasons too, vegans and vegetarians for example. As long as your core diet consists of reasonable portions with enough food groups to give you all the nutrients your body needs, and you have the occasional treat (and be honest with yourself, is it really just occasional, or are you gorging a whole packet of biscuits down your face every time your favourite TV programme is on?) then you will be fine.

So why is there so much confusion about which diet is best, and why is there so much misinformation and lack of real knowledge about weight and health? I don't know, I wish I did. I'd probably be a very rich man! I suspect it's due to peoples innate ability to dismiss anything that would involve effort and reach for that quick fix instead. So before I tell you exactly what constitutes a healthy diet, we should dispel a few of the myths and misunderstandings that some of you may have about food, weight and health.

Do I need to count calories?

Counting calories seems to by a mainstay of many fad diets and fat clubs, with devotees getting out the calculator before every meal, slavishly adding up every calorie in every morsel of food just in case they go over their allocated amount on a day they are not allowed to.

This is extremely simplistic at best, and unfortunately the importance of calories is more complex than that. Fortunately once you know the basics, then using calories to lose weight and maintain a healthy body fat level becomes much easier.

The recommended calorie intake for adult men is approximately 2,500 per day, whilst for adult women it is approximately 1,950. This is an average number that men and women need to survive and function with a basic sedentary lifestyle. If you consume more calories than this number without somehow burning it off, then you will gain body fat (and therefore weight). If you consume slightly less than this number or burn off more than you consume through activity or exercise, then you will burn up body fat. Simple so far, right?

What many people fail to take into account however is that very active lifestyles, active jobs and exercise all have an effect on this number, and those who have such a lifestyle will need more calories just to function. Athletes for example can significantly increase, even double the number of calories they need per day without gaining any body fat, because they need far more energy than the average Joe couch potato, and all that excess energy is used up. This is why many people find that they have a need to eat a lot more once they start exercising.

What is also important to remember is what happens if you consume too few calories by skipping meals or not eating enough due to some half baked diet plan you found somewhere. This is where you essentially start to starve yourself. Many fad diets do not come close to providing people with the amount of calories they need to function, and yes they lose weight, but it is not 'healthy weight' they are losing, as muscle will atrophy or waste away too, and they will not have enough energy to get through the day or maintain a healthy lifestyle.

Other factors too have an effect on the amount of calories you will need during the day, your age, height and other biological factors all play their part. That is why it is important to determine your own individual caloric needs. Remember that basic number of approximately 2,500 per day for men and approximately 1,950 for women. Now think of your age, your actual levels of exercise, the amount of muscle you have on you, your activity throughout an average day (sitting at a desk as opposed to working on a building site for example), all of these play a part.

Now, the most important piece of information I can give you is that it isn't just the number of calories you have to count, but the type of calories too. This basically means quality, not quantity. Imagine one woman who eats slightly below her allocated calorie intake every day, but every single one of those calories come from chocolate, fast food and alcohol. Now imagine another woman who eats slightly more than her allocated daily intake, but those calories come from lean meat, vegetables and rice or pasta. That second woman is getting all the right nutrients and as a result will be much, much healthier. I know many of you won't fall into these extreme categories as most people fall somewhere in the middle, but they are still useful as examples.

So, what are these good calories then? To answer that, now you need to understand a little bit about the food you are eating.

What foods do I eat in a healthy diet?

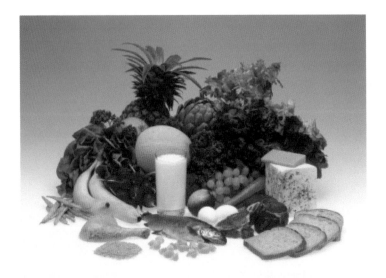

There are a thousand and one diet and recipe books out there, from celebrity chefs to some chancer who picks up a wok. Everyone and their aunt has an opinion on what to eat, when to eat it and what is and isn't good for you, and perhaps the worst offenders are those fad diet articles in women's magazines. I'm not surprised so many patients of mine are so confused as to what constitutes a healthy diet.

So instead of giving you a load of recipes or a list of foods that you should avoid at all costs, I'm going to tell you a little bit about the types of food you are putting into your mouth and how to eat a healthy, balanced diet to maintain a healthy lifestyle. Don't worry, it isn't as complicated as it sounds.

Top Tip! A healthy diet should contain a lot of fresh fruit and vegetables, some starchy carbs , some protein, a little bit of dairy products and a small, limited amount of fat and sugar.

One of the most important factors to remember is that your diet should contain a variety of foods from a range of sources. Different nutrients are present in different food stuffs and in different quantities, so by getting a wide variety of food, that way you can ensure that your body is getting all the correct nutrients. Hey, I've effectively just given you free reign to go wild at a buffet! Good times! But don't forget, it isn't just the quantity, it is the quality and type of food you are eating too!

As I'm sure you are aware, there are different types of foods, or food groups, and it is important to get the balance between each group right for every meal. As long as you get the balance right, and you vary the foods within those groups from day to day, you will be eating a healthy and varied diet. By making portion sizes relative to your calorific needs, you will lose or maintain a healthy level of body fat whilst allowing for the occasional treat. It really is that simple.

Fruit and vegetables.

The first group is fresh fruit and vegetables. Obvious really isn't it? This is arguably one of the most important groups but for some reason one that many people struggle with. Fruit and vegetables should make up roughly a third of your daily diet and the current recommended guidelines in the UK state that you should have at least 5 portions a day. Personally, I would argue that number is far too low and should be considered as a minimum. It was a number put in place for a society that seems scared of going into the fruit and vegetable aisle of the supermarkets and for children who think a potato is a carrot and crisps are vegetables. Basically more is better, and I would double the recommended number at least. Don't worry, it is much easier than it sounds. The Japanese government for example recommends up to 17 portions a day!

> Myth buster! It's too hard to eat 5 a day! No it isn't! It's easy! Have a piece of fruit plus some fruit juice in the morning along with your breakfast, snack on another piece of fruit mid morning, and then put lettuce and a cucumber on your sandwich for lunch. There's five right there, and you haven't even got to your main meal yet!

So why are fruit and vegetables so important? The answer is quite simple and self explanatory really, the nutrients inside them are essential to a healthy, balanced diet and can reduce the risk of many long term chronic health conditions such as heart disease, high blood pressure, type II diabetes and even certain cancers.

Different fruits and vegetables have a wide range of vitamins, minerals, fibre, antioxidants and other phytonutrients that all have a benefit to your health. That is why it is important to eat a wide range of different fruit and vegetables in order to get as wide a range of all these nutrients as possible.

Starchy foods.

This second group consists of starchy foods such as bread, rice, pasta and potatoes. These are the main source of carbohydrate, or carbs, and are important to not only a healthy, balanced diet but to living a healthy lifestyle too. I cannot stress this enough, carbohydrates are essential, regardless of all the ridiculous fad diets and myths that have been circulating for years now.

> Myth buster! Do I need to cut out carbs completely to lose weight? No you don't! That's Rubbish! Low carb or no carb diets do you more harm than good. Cutting out carbohydrate sources such as rice and pasta completely means you miss out on the energy that these food sources supply, as well as all the other nutrients. By not supplying your body with carbohydrate, you are forcing your body to use up protein for energy instead, which will waste away your muscles and tissue, and put a lot of stress on the kidneys and heart, leading eventually to heart and acute kidney problems.

Potatoes, rice, pasta or other starchy foods should again make up roughly another third of your daily dietary intake. It is a good idea wherever possible to choose wholegrain varieties because of the extra nutrients such as fibre, although this certainly is not essential all the time as long as you get those nutrients elsewhere.

As well as a range of nutrients such as fibre, calcium, iron and vitamins, starchy foods contain carbohydrates, which is where we will get most of our energy from. If you want to do any exercise or live an active lifestyle, you simply will not be able to cope without energy. It doesn't matter whether you run, lift weights, play a sport or go swimming, the more exercise you do, the more carbohydrates you will need to supply that energy source.

Meat and Fish.

Meat and fish should be the next thing you put on your plate. You've already used up two thirds of your total daily intake with fresh fruit and vegetables and starchy carbohydrates, so meat and fish should be a little less than a third. Remember, you don't have to be completely exact with these measurements as long as they roughly approximate what you eat daily, they are just there as a basic guide.

Meat and fish are rich in protein as well as many other nutrients such as iron, and it is essential that you include this as part of a healthy diet. Vegans and vegetarians must obtain the nutrients from elsewhere, such as beans and pulses or soya, but for the rest of us, chicken, pork, beef, or a variety of fish should form part of a balanced healthy diet. No, that doesn't mean chicken nuggets are okay!

The type of meat you include in your diet and the way you cook it is essential. When cooking the meat, remember to remove any excess fat or skin, and grill or oven cook the meat rather than frying it in oil, this will reduce the fat content in the meat you do have. You may have heard too much red meat can be bad for you, and that is partly true. A diet that consists of a large proportion of red meat (pork or beef) and processed meat (such as sausages, ham, bacon and so on) can increase your risk of certain types of cancer. Furthermore, red and processed meat are much more likely to have higher levels of saturated fat, which can raise cholesterol levels. However, that isn't to say you can't have them at all. Limit your red meat intake to say once a week, maybe twice a week once in a while, and have no more than 70 grams of processed meat a day (that's just a couple of sausages or two rashers of bacon). I will never deny you that beef Sunday dinner or a bacon sandwich the morning after the night before, that would be impractical, and probably cruel too. I'm just saying limit it so you aren't eating those food types every day. Lean meat such as chicken or turkey or a variety of oily fishes, which also contain great doses of Omega 3, should make up the bulk of your weekly meat intake.

Eggs can also be included in this category, and yes I know that it isn't a slab of meat, but eggs are a great source of protein too, as well as a number of vitamins. So throw in the occasional scrambled egg for breakfast instead of sausages, or have a vegetable omelette instead, as part of a varied diet, they can be a great way of ensuring you get the protein your body needs. Unfortunately guys, I can't recommend drinking a pint of raw eggs and then running round the garden singing the Rocky theme tune, sorry. You have to make sure they're cooked thoroughly!

When cooking the meat, remember to remove any excess fat or skin, and grill or oven cook the meat rather than frying it in oil, this will reduce the fat content in the meat you do have.

Dairy foods.

In moderation, dairy products such as milk and cheese can be valuable sources of protein, calcium and a variety of other vitamins and minerals. But dairy products can also contain a large amount of fat, and should only be a relatively small part of your daily diet. Don't worry about it too much, because it is important to get some rather than none at all. You can help limit the fat content by choosing lower fat milks , limiting your cheese (which can also have too much salt) and low fat margarine instead of butter.

Fat and Sugar.

These should obviously be a small part of your daily diet and on the whole, limited to the occasional treat. It goes without saying that eating too much fatty foods will make us fat. The more fatty foods you eat, the more body fat and weight you will gain and the more you will suffer from weight related health problems. It's obvious.

However, a tiny bit of the right type of fat in our diet is fine, and is actually healthy as it can provide the body with essential fatty acids and provide a mechanism for absorbing certain nutrients such as fibre.

So how do you know what fats to eat and how much? Well for that you need to know some basic facts. There are two types of fat, saturated and non saturated. In terms of calorie levels, they are generally both the same, so eating too much of either will make you gain weight. However, saturated fats should be avoided wherever possible. This is the type of fat found in the fat cuts of meat, the fatty bits of bacon, processed meats such as sausages, lard and butter, hard cheese, ice cream, pastries and so on. The saturated fats found in these foods will not only make you gain body fat, but will raise your cholesterol levels over time, and lead to a variety of health problems, not least of which is heart disease. Unsaturated fat on the other hand is found naturally in oily fish, nuts and seeds and so on, and can also be found in some of the better olive oils, sunflower oil and spreads.

> Myth buster! Low fat or reduced fat foods aren't always healthy! Remember, the reduced fat item may still be high in fat, and the fat is often replaced with sugar so may be even higher in calories than the high fat version! Check the nutrition labels carefully.

Obviously it is much better to choose unsaturated fats wherever possible and use them in a small portion of your daily diet. Doing this will actually reduce your cholesterol levels if they are high, or at the least keep them balanced, and provide your body with the healthy levels of fat it needs. If you must have foods with saturated fats, then try to limit them as much as possible and use tricks such as cutting the fatty bits off bacon and meat to limit it even further.

Sugar is most people's Achilles heel when it comes to eating a healthy diet. Who doesn't enjoy the odd biscuit when they curl up in front of the TV? Sweets, chocolate, fizzy drinks, they are a constant in most of our lives, and the majority of people eat significantly more than is recommended for a healthy, balanced diet. I have even met people whose primary diet consisted of more than 90% of large amounts of sugary food and drinks, with the other 10% being microwave meals, sausage rolls and pasties and pretty much nothing else, and then wondered why they had to come to me with a range of health problems! I kid you not!

The thing with sugar is that when it is found in foods, it often comes hand in hand with calories too, and very little else in the way of nutrients. So when a large proportion of our diet consists of these foods, we deny ourselves a variety of nutrients and pile on the calories, which isn't good for our health or our body fat levels!

But as I have always said to my patients who ask for diet advice, and to myself when I practice what I preach, no one should deny themselves the occasional treat. Life is far too short to do that and food is after all there to be enjoyed! It can actually be healthy from a mental health and stress point of view to allow yourself these treats. Just don't allow them to become too regular, or to dominate an unbalanced diet. Limit them to a treat, make them a tiny part of what is on the whole a predominantly healthy, balanced diet, and get enough exercise to balance the extra calories and you will be absolutely fine!

> Myth buster! It is too expensive to eat a healthy diet! Rubbish. I know food in general is shooting up in price, but you can still get all the staples you need for a healthy diet for the same as or even less than a week's worth of microwave meals, sugary snacks and especially takeaways.

So when you are doing your weekly shopping and planning your healthy diet, just remember, at least an approximate third of your total daily intake should be as wide a variety of fresh fruit and vegetables as you can get. Another third should be from starchy foods full of carbohydrates for energy, try and use some wholegrain alternatives too. A good portion of meat and fish, especially lean meat and oily fish for protein should make up almost all of the rest of your dietary intake with a small amount of dairy products to complete the healthy, balanced diet. Limited amounts of sugar and fats can be limited as occasional treats. It is not necessary to have each food group present in every single meal (although your main meals of the day should contain at least three), as long as throughout the day you get the balance and variety right.

So what are all these vital nutrients?

Now you know the basic food groups that make up a healthy, balanced meal, it is important you understand exactly what these separate components contain and why it is important that they are included in your daily diet. It is easy sometimes to talk about all these different nutrients and forget that it can sometimes be overwhelming for people to have words like protein and antioxidants thrown at them without an explanation, so that is what I'll do here.

Carbohydrates.

Carbohydrates are a vital source of energy for the body, and quite simply we need it to maintain a healthy lifestyle. The process behind it is relatively straightforward. Once you have eaten that big bowl of pasta or rice, the carbohydrates inside it break down into sugar, specifically known as glucose, fructose and galactose. These sugars then break down even further and get absorbed into the body, either to be used as energy straight away, or stored in the muscles in the form of glycogen. Now this is the part where all those ridiculous myths about low carb diets sprang up from. Any excess glycogen that cannot be stored in the muscles or used up will be stored as fat instead. But that does not mean that you should cut them out completely to avoid the fat storage part of the process, as cutting out carbohydrates completely and replacing them with fat and protein only can and will have negative health effects. That is why it is important to ensure that your daily starch intake is roughly a third of your whole daily diet, or you use up any extra you eat by exercising. But remember, by exercising properly and increasing the levels of glycogen your body needs, you are increasing the levels of calories you will need to consume in order to function at that level. That's the reason you so often hear of athletes competing at a high level eating huge mounds of food constantly, and why all those people who eat the same amount but do no exercise just get fat.

Now just to make it slightly more complex, if you will excuse the pun, there are two types of carbohydrate, simple and complex. Simple carbs are absorbed and used up by the body very quickly, whilst complex carbs are absorbed much more slowly and provide a slow release of energy. Simple carbs are found in fruit, energy drinks and so on, and complex carbs are what people tend to traditionally think of, that is pasta, breads, rice and potatoes. That is why if I get a patient whose blood sugars drop suddenly, the old trick of a cup of a certain energy drink and then some toast works really well, because the simple carbs in the drink raise the blood sugar and give the patient a short term burst of energy, and the complex carbs in the toast keep the blood sugars stable with a slow release of energy over a longer period. The same principle can apply to athletes or anyone going about their average active lifestyle. The complex carbs in a healthy diet will give you a slow release of energy throughout the day, providing that you eat say some porridge for breakfast, have a sandwich or jacket potato for lunch, and some pasta for dinner. You have a stable, slow release energy source there to keep you going throughout the day. However, if you are feeling a little low or tired, or you suddenly need a boost for a burst of exercise, then fresh fruit or energy drinks (in limited amounts) will supply you with the simple carbs you need for that rapid burst of energy. See? It really isn't as scary as all those fad diets made out, is it?

Carbohydrate management in diabetes.

It is essential that people who have any type of diabetes manage their food consumption well and eat a healthy balanced diet. An important part of any healthy diet is starchy carbohydrates, but it is much more important for diabetics as they help to maintain a stable blood glucose level.

Many diabetics have had adverse side effects whilst trying out certain low carb or no carb fad diets, without quite realising why or what is happening, and whilst it can be beneficial to slightly cut down on carbohydrate intake if you are trying to lose body fat and are eating too much, diabetics in particular have to be careful that they do not cut out too much. Carbohydrates are essential. That is a simple, and undeniable fact. Low or no carb diets can be harmful. I really don't know how to say that any simpler.

For type 1 diabetics, or type 2 diabetics who require insulin, then carbohydrate counting will be a term you may have come across. This is an extremely important, but sometimes confusing term that you need to become familiar with.

All it is, is a method of matching the amount of carbohydrates in your everyday diet with the amount of insulin you need to take, basically a method of maintaining your blood glucose levels. To master this technique, you will need to understand about how carbohydrates interact with your body and be very familiar with your own individual insulin requirements. Constant monitoring of your blood glucose is essential, and you will need to adjust either your insulin or your carbohydrate intake as needed. There is no one size fits all rule to this, as every person is completely individual and will have different requirements. The best guidance I can give you in this book is speak to a healthcare professional such as a diabetes nurse, who will be able to guide you based on your own individual needs.

Protein.

Protein is primarily obtained from a variety of meat, eggs and fish sources, but can also be found in some fruits, pulses, nuts, milk, and wholegrain cereals to a limited extent. There are so many myths and misunderstandings about protein, especially amongst guys who think by downing 2 pints of a ridiculous protein shake will make them look like a bodybuilder overnight, or those insane fad diets that promise you a beach body if you eat nothing but protein!

The fact is it is a simple, but essential nutrient for our bodies to function, without it our muscles and cells would not be able to grow, repair or even maintain themselves. Protein is made up of amino acids, and these are broken down during digestion into polypeptides, which then provide the amino acids to replace those lost during the day as the body uses up its protein stores. A number of these are called essential amino acids, simply meaning that our body does not produce them naturally, so it is essential that we get them from our diet, this is where the term 'complete protein source' comes from, it simply means that the source provides all the essential amino acids your body needs, and can come from any meat, fish, eggs, or even some dairy products. This just means that other smaller sources of protein such as tofu, pulses or rice are incomplete protein sources, and must be eaten together in a wider variety to get the same level of essential amino acids. This is why it is essential that vegetarians and vegans, especially if they weight train or are pregnant, pay close attention to their diet and ensure they get enough sources of protein.

It is undeniable that without protein, our bodies would not be able to function, it really is as simple as that; but it is it's applications for exercise, specifically for strength training, where people tend to start thinking of it as a nutrient they should be getting in their diets. The truth is it should be an essential part of everyone's diet. Protein deficiency, especially in risk groups such as young children and pregnant women, can be a real problem and lead to a wide variety of malnutrition related health problems, often exacerbated by the fact that it is often overlooked.

Those who lead active lifestyles or a lot of exercise however, particularly strength exercises, will need to get enough protein in their diets to supply the energy they need, and to repair and build muscle and tissue.

The amount of protein each person needs will be very dependent on individual circumstance. The average is 46 grams per day for women aged 19 - 70, or 56 grams a day for men of the same age. That is about 6 - 7 ounces of meat and a glass of milk or two in real money, but this can easily be affected by individual energy and exercise needs, body composition and weight, carbohydrate intake, how much strength or muscular training they do and so on. Athletes, those with larger amounts of muscle mass or women who are pregnant, will also require greater levels of protein.

Protein in exercise.

When exercising, protein is needed to repair and build the muscles after use, as well as provide a source of energy alongside carbohydrates. Strength training activities and sports such as weightlifting will require a greater amount of protein in a daily balanced diet than those who live sedentary lifestyles. It is common sense really, someone who lifts a lot of weights will need a lot more energy and muscle repairing and building protein than someone who slobs in front of the TV all day.

When you exercise, particularly lifting weights, you damage your muscle fibres. That isn't as bad as it sounds, the process of repairing the muscle is what helps it to grow bigger and stronger. Protein actually aids the repair of this damage, and aids muscle recovery and adaptation too, which will allow your muscles to change and grow.

Endurance athletes such as runners and swimmers may think that they don't need protein, as their primary form of training is aerobic, or cardiovascular. Whilst it is true that they may not need as much protein as a bodybuilder, they still need to repair and build the muscles they do use, so an increase in the protein part of their diet will still be beneficial.

It is a topic of debate as to exactly how much extra protein you need when you exercise or weight train, with actual measurements varying from country to country and opinion to opinion. However, almost all theories agree that protein consumption does need to increase based on very individual age, weight and body composition and level, type and rate of exercise, and that these extra levels can easily be met through diet alone without the need for supplements.

It is also important to remember that in general, an increase in the amount of protein you consume in your daily diet can be extremely beneficial if you exercise or weight train, but it is important to increase this alongside an increase in your carbohydrate and calorie intake too, and it is important to counter this with your level of activity. Basically eat as much as you need to provide your body with fuel, no more, no less, as too much protein can have harmful side effects.

Too much protein?

Generally in Western countries, people consume more protein than they actually need for their level of activity, as it is a nutrient found easily in abundance in many different food sources. Perhaps the worst culprits are those men who fall for the 'look at me' adverts of some huge bodybuilder holding a wonder protein drink that promises a body that certain Austrian powerhouse would be proud of. I see this all the time at the gym, men of all shapes and sizes gulping back huge amounts of protein shakes before strutting around the gym, and usually after training incorrectly too. I seriously want to bang my head against a brick wall sometimes.

> Myth buster! If I weight train I have to take protein supplements to get big. Absolute rubbish. The truth is you will only gain muscle mass by putting in the hard work, and you don't need supplements at all. All the protein your body needs can be gained from eating a healthy, balanced diet based around your weight and training requirements? Why have a protein shake when a nice big bowl of chicken salad is the alternative?

Now in small quantities, eating a bit more protein that your body needs will not have much of a harmful effect other than making you pile on a few pounds. Protein does contribute to calorie intake, so unless you burn it off and use the protein, your body fat levels will increase.

However in larger quantities and over an extended period of time, too much protein can actually harm your body. Yes I'm talking specifically to you guys at the gym here, or those of you who looked at the high protein diet and thought it was a good idea! What can happen, is over time your body can build up ketones. These build up when your body does not get the energy it needs from carbs or sugar, but too much protein and fatty acids. Ketones are toxic to your body, and you will normally have no trouble excreting them, but if they are allowed to build up through too much protein or a high protein, low carb diet, then this alters the PH level of your urine making it slightly acidic (you may notice a much stronger smell). This will put unnecessary stress on the kidneys as it works harder to flush them out, and increase the risk of kidney stones and even kidney damage over an extended period of time. This process can also lead to dehydration, loss of muscle mass and bad breath. Are those protein shakes looking as good now? I didn't think so.

Vitamins and minerals.

Vitamins are an essential nutrient contained in fresh fruit and vegetables as well as other food sources such as meat and cod liver oil for example, each have recommended daily amounts and deficiencies in certain vitamins can have serious long term health effects, with scurvy and rickets being amongst the most well known. Although supplements are available, a balanced diet with a wide range of fresh fruit and vegetables is sufficient to gain your daily needs, and overdosing can occur with supplements on top of a healthy diet. An extensive knowledge of which vitamin does what is not really necessary, just a basic knowledge of what they do and which foods they are found in, contained in the table below, will often be enough for most people to ensure they are eating enough.

Vitamins.

Vitamins are something that almost everyone has heard of, usually through a supplement advert on the TV or a health food shop trying to palm the latest wonder pill on you. The truth is, vitamins are an essential nutrient found in a variety of foods, and as long as we eat a healthy, varied diet, we will get the full range of vitamins that we need. It is essential that we get all the necessary vitamins, because vitamin deficiency is a real problem and can lead to a wide variety of ailments and illnesses. Supplements are usually only necessary in medical conditions or when other factors come into play that means that you literally cannot consume the right foods or drinks to get the vitamins you need. For most of us, supplements aren't necessary.

There are a wide variety of different vitamins, and they are found in an even wider range of foods and all have different benefits.

Vitamin A:

Commonly found in a range of leafy vegetables, carrots, pumpkins, citrus coloured fruits, spinach and liver, and is useful for vision, our immune system, bone, skin and cellular health and is a good source of antioxidants. A deficiency in vitamin A can lead to Keratomalacia and Nyctalopia or 'night blindness'. It is the reason we were all told as kids that carrots helped us see in the dark!

Vitamin B1:

Commonly found in high protein sources such as pork, liver and eggs, as well as a range of vegetables, potatoes and brown rice. It is also sometimes referred to as Thiamine, and can help to prevent Thiamine deficiency ailments of the nervous system, such as beriberi or Wernicke - Korsakoff syndrome.

Vitamin B2:

Vitamin B2, or Riboflavin, is found in bananas and a range of dairy products such as milk, as well as some green vegetables such as green beans. It is essential in preventing Ariboflavinosis.

Vitamin B3:

Also known as niacin, it is found in high protein sources such as meat, fish, eggs and nuts, as well as a wide range of vegetables and mushrooms. Vitamin B3 deficiency can lead to a condition known as Pellagra, which is a pretty nasty ailment that can present with skin lesions, diarrhoea, weakness, dementia and others.

Vitamin B5:

Found in most foods in small doses, but especially green vegetables such as broccoli.

Vitamin B6:

Found in a wide range of meats, nuts, vegetables and bananas, a vitamin B6 deficiency can lead to anaemia and peripheral neuropathy.

Vitamin B7:

Found in eggs, liver, peanuts and a range of vegetables, a lack of vitamin b9 is a cause of dermatitis and enteritis.

Vitamin B9:

Otherwise known as folic acid, this vitamin is found in a range of leafy vegetables, pasta, breads, cereals and liver. It is important for a variety of reasons, but a deficiency during pregnancy has been associated with a number of birth defects.

Vitamin B12:

Found in meat, fat and some dairy products, it is important in preventing megaloblastic anaemia.

Vitamin C:

The vitamin most people are familiar with, also known as ascorbic acid. It is found in a huge variety of fruits and vegetables, particularly citrus fruits such as oranges. It is a great source of antioxidants, is a natural antihistamine and is useful to boost the immune system and preventing scurvy, which is a vitamin C deficiency disease.

Vitamin D:

This is commonly known as the sunshine vitamin, because you get it from sunlight. It is present naturally in some foods, but not many, and not in great quantities. Fish, such as tuna, mackerel, salmon and herring contain small amounts, as do shitake mushrooms. Vitamin D is useful in preventing rickets and osteomalacia, which is a softening of the bones.

Vitamin E:

Commonly found in a wide variety of fruits and vegetables. It is a great source of antioxidants, can help muscle growth by acting as an enzymatic regulator and prevents the oxidisation of polyunsaturated fatty acids. Vitamin E deficiencies can lead to neuropathy and myopathy (muscular weakness), skeletal myopathy, ataxia and immune response impairment.

Vitamin K:

Vitamin K is found in a range of vegetables, particularly green leafy vegetables such as spinach, Kale, broccoli and cabbage, and is essential for bone growth and health. A deficiency is rare in most diets, but can lead to bleeding disorders and heavy menstrual bleeding in women.

This is not an extensive list of each vitamins sources or uses, but will give you a basic understanding of why each one is necessary. Remember, a healthy, varied diet will get you most if not all the vitamins you need without the need for any supplements. If you eat a good healthy diet and take supplements as well, be careful of overdosing on them too.

Minerals.

Mineral nutrients are often less well known than vitamins, but are equally as important. Minerals such as calcium, potassium, iron, sodium and magnesium, amongst others all play a vital role in health, and as a staff nurse I spend a lot of time examining the exact balance of these nutrients via blood samples to determine what is wrong with a patient and what I can do to help fix it. Again it is not necessary to have an in depth medical knowledge to understand how an excess or deficiency of these minerals can affect your health, nor is it necessary to know all of them, but it is important to have a basic understanding of what some of the most important minerals are and what they do, so you can make informed choices about your dietary intake and eat a healthy, balanced diet.

Potassium.

Potassium is found in many foods such as meat and fish, and a lot of fruit and vegetables such as bananas, prunes, avocadoes and many more besides, works with sodium to help maintain the body's natural fluid and electrolyte balance, and is important in nerve and muscular function, specifically muscle contraction. It is recommended that the levels of Potassium and Sodium consumed daily should be roughly equal, and studies have shown that an optimal intake of potassium can reduce the risk of hypertension and stroke. It is important to note however that relatively common conditions such as dehydration and diarrhoea without taking steps to replace potassium levels can easily lead to potassium depletion and hypokolemia (low potassium), causing muscle weakness, impaired kidney function and even cardiac arrhythmia if left untreated. Potassium excretion is controlled by the kidneys, so it is important to consider also that anyone suffering from acute kidney diseases have to be careful to observe a strict diet so they do not get too much, which can lead to hyperkalemia (high potassium), and heart problems. It's a pretty delicate balancing act!

Sodium.

Sodium is the other half to this delicate balancing act. And by sodium, or sodium chloride I basically mean salt. Sodium intake is traditionally extremely high in many Western countries, far exceeding the recommended daily amounts, and is a leading cause of developing high blood pressure or hypertension, and like Potassium, sodium excretion is controlled by the kidneys, so excess amounts can lead to oedema or fluid retention. Yet by the same account, sodium is necessary for life and the basic functioning of a healthy body, so how much is too much? There is a huge amount of debate on the use of salt, basically boiling down to should you use it or shouldn't you? Well the truth of the matter is it depends on the type of salt. The recommended daily amount is no more than 6 grams a day for an adult, that's just one simple teaspoon of the stuff, no more, so check how much you are shaking onto your chips the next time you reach for it! The reality is that sodium is present naturally in most of the foods we eat, from bread and cereals to bacon and fish, and the levels of unrefined salt in processed package food is much, much higher still. So by eating a varied diet we can easily get our recommended daily amounts. Quite frankly there is no need to have refined table salt at all, and often it is the use of this to flavour food, on top of the amount of naturally occurring sodium in the foods we eat that pushes our sodium levels above what they should be. If you have to use salt in cooking then use unrefined sea salt, which is much higher in other trace minerals as the refining process hasn't removed them.

Calcium.

Calcium is another essential mineral, especially in children as they are developing, but just as important in adults too. I'm sure many of you know that Calcium is essential in the formation and strength of healthy bones and teeth, but did you know that it is also important in reducing the risk of osteoporosis and in regulating muscle contraction?

Many of you will know that calcium is found in dairy products. Milk especially has long been considered to be one of the most important sources of calcium, and this is true, but calcium can also be found in fish, sesame seeds, some fruit, almonds, figs, soya and some dark green, leafy vegetables. So those of you who are vegans need not miss out!

The recommended daily amount of calcium for adults between 19 - 70 is 1000 mg per day. Obviously children, teenagers, the elderly and pregnant women will have different RDA's dependent of specific needs. This basically boils down to three or four portions of dairy products a day, since I know none of you will go out and measure exactly 1000 mg! One portion can be roughly 200 ml of milk (how many cups of tea you can get out of that depends on how milky you like it) or a small pot of yoghurt for example. I'm not going to suggest you go out and measure exact amounts out, that would be daft, I just want to impress on you the importance of using common sense and having at least this amount as a minimum daily. Don't worry, I'm not going to deny you that extra cup of milky tea after a long day if you go over the RDA! When choosing your sources of calcium however, try to choose skimmed or semi skimmed milks or no sugar, unsweetened yoghurts (especially if they contain other things like probiotics), and try to limit the fatty/salty cheeses, especially if you are trying to decrease your body fat levels.

Iron.

Iron is yet another mineral that is vital for life and an essential part of a healthy diet. It exists in the haemoglobin of our red blood cells and assists in the oxygenation of the blood before being utilised by other tissues, specifically muscle.

Dietary sources of iron consist of heam iron and non heam iron, basically meaning iron that comes from animals (which once had red blood cells, hence the term 'heam'), or plants, which did not, and the sources are varied. The most concentrated sources are found in red meat and offal such as beef, pork and liver. Chicken, turkey and fish, although not containing quite as high levels as red meat, are still excellent sources of iron. Other sources are green leafy vegetables such as spinach or pak choi, pulses, nuts, cereals and whole grains, although these aren't as easily absorbed by the body, they are still useful, particularly for vegetarians.

The recommended daily amount of iron is 8.7 mg for men aged 18 - 50 and 14.8 mg for women of the same age. Although be aware that this does change for different age groups or pregnant women. Iron deficiency is a huge problem, especially around the world, with the World Health Organisation naming it as one of the most common nutritional deficiencies.

A lack of iron in your diet can over time result in a condition known as iron deficiency anaemia. This happens over a relatively long period of time, and by the time it occurs there has usually been a prolonged period of an iron deficient diet, leaving the body in a negative balance. You don't need to have developed full iron deficiency anaemia to feel the effects of low levels of iron, which can lead to feeling tired, unable to concentrate or sometimes feelings of dizziness, a general lack of energy or lethargy, and a pale skin colour. Certain groups such as infants, teenage girls, menstruating women, pregnant women, vegetarians and vegans and the elderly, especially if they are malnourished, are at more risk of developing this than others, or at the very least feel some of the tiring effects of low iron levels at certain times. Iron deficiency anaemia can be corrected over time with a mixture of diet and supplements, depending on the severity, but it is much better to ensure that you are eating enough iron in your diet in the first place. So pile up that meat and dark green leafy veg on your plate!

Fibre.

Fibre is another vital part of our diet, but again is one that is often ignored. The recommended daily amount is at least 18 grams, and a significant number of people quite simply do not get enough of it. Fibre is basically found in foods that are made from plants. Sound simple? Good, it is. Wheat, corn, bran, potato skins, fruits and vegetables (their skins as well as their insides), nuts and so on are all great sources of fibre, and foods made of these base ingredients, such as cereals, wholegrain pasta and wholemeal bread are too. (No, crisps don't really count because they are made from potatoes, sorry).

There are two types of fibre, soluble and insoluble, and both have different but equally important benefits. Don't worry though, most foods that contain fibre will have a mixture of both to a greater or lesser degree, so again, by eating that wonderful varied diet, you will be sure to get both.

There are many benefits to an optimum dietary fibre intake. Fibre is essential in maintaining a healthy gastrointestinal tract and preventing digestive problems. Basically, it keeps you regular and stops you getting constipated or having diarrhoea. Soluble fibre can be digested, and can help to reduce your cholesterol, whilst insoluble fibre is the stuff that can't be digested, and instead helps move everything else through your digestive system. On top of this, it also helps your body absorb and extract the essential nutrients it needs from food as it passes through your bowels, by making sure that it passes through at the right speed, and in turn helps regulate blood sugar and improves glucose tolerance which is essential for diabetics. It also reduces the risk of certain cancers. If you still needed any more encouragement to include a healthy fibre intake into your diet, it also makes you feel fuller for longer, helping weight management.

It is also important to stress however that as important as fibre is, it is essential to drink plenty of fluids alongside it, and to not consume too much fibre or too quickly. Eating too much can lead to constipation, whilst eating too much too quickly can cause cramps, bloating and wind. So basically fibre is an essential part of your diet, you need it. Just stick to the recommended daily amounts and eat regularly throughout the day, not all at once!

Antioxidants.

Antioxidants have had a lot of weird and wonderful claims attributed to them over the years, from anti ageing properties to supercharging your immune system so you will never be ill or even turning you into a superhero akin to a comic book character. It is important to note that there is currently a lot of debate and research on this subject, so no claim like this should be taken as fact just yet. Those who read some of the articles in the plethora of women's magazines out there, or have seen the labels on certain fruit juices will be familiar with some of these claims, but for all these wild assertions there is almost as much widespread confusion as to what exactly they are.

The truth is the term itself is slightly misleading. Antioxidants is a bit of an umbrella term, used to describe a range of vitamins, minerals and nutrients that repair and protect cell damage from free radicals.

Without wanting to descend into a Chemistry class, free radicals are basically formed when atoms split due to a weak electron bond, they then go on to attack other healthy molecules and form a chain reaction. This does happen naturally within the body during metabolism, and normally the body can handle it in small amounts because we naturally get certain amounts of free radicals in a basic diet. However, modern lifestyles that expose the body to pollution, low level radiation, herbicides, poor diets and perhaps more significant than anything else, cigarette smoke, can lead to a huge increase in free radical production, and this increases with age.

So what do antioxidants do to stop this? Basically they neutralise the destructive chain reaction by adding electrons into the molecules and stop the electrons from being lost, therefore stopping the molecule from becoming a free radical.

I'm sorry, I know this chemistry stuff can get a bit heavy. But it is essential to know exactly why antioxidants are important. By stopping the chain reaction and the damage from free radicals, many experts say that antioxidants can help stop or at least reduce the effect free radicals have on chronic diseases such as atherosclerosis, certain cancers, arthritis and so on, and even improving the effectiveness of your immune system, leading to common illnesses such as colds, sore throats and other infections; and hey, if someone at some point in the future does happen to prove that they slow the aging process too, then I doubt anyone would complain!

Basically to ensure you get enough of these antioxidants, you need to ensure that you are eating a wide range of fruit and vegetables, and plenty of them too. Beta carotene, vitamin C and vitamin E are three vitamins that have higher levels of antioxidants than others, and these can be found in a variety of brightly coloured fruits and vegetables. Beta carotene and carotenoids for example are in abundance in carrots, corn, green peppers, spinach, broccoli, potatoes, kale, mangoes, apricots, watermelon and many other fruit and vegetables. Vitamin C is abundant in many citrus fruits, berries, red, green or yellow peppers, strawberries, tomatoes and grapefruits, whilst vitamin E is often found in broccoli, turnips, nuts, papaya, pumpkins and many other fruits and vegetables. Zinc and Selenium, found in tuna, beef, poultry, seafood, grain and dairy products are also said to contain antioxidants. The list isn't meant to be exhaustive, just give you a brief example of where you can find the vitamins and nutrients where you can get your fill of antioxidants, so get eating!

What about chocolate?

There is absolutely nothing wrong with having the occasional chocolate bar, or pizza, or takeaway or anything else for that matter. Yes, you did hear me right, this is a diet that allows chocolate, and I am a staff nurse advocating chocolate and other treats as part of a healthy, balanced diet. The secret is moderation. If the large bulk of your diet is healthy, varied and contains all the nutrients your body needs, plus you get regular exercise to counter the extra calories, then quite frankly it doesn't really matter if you want a chocolate bar once in a while or you fancy having a lazy day and ordering a takeaway! It's fine, go ahead, there's no guilt involved either!

I'm not going to tell you exactly how much you can and can't have, or tell you that you are only allowed one treat day once every two months on a Wednesday because that is what your plan dictates. I can't do that. It is ridiculous to even try. What constitutes a treat in moderation is totally down to you as an individual, how much of a healthy, varied diet you eat normally, how much exercise you do and what your health and fitness goals are. Only you can determine that.

What I want to get across to you is that you shouldn't feel guilty for having the occasional treat. Life is too short to deny yourself and food is a wonderful thing to enjoy, especially when its covered in chocolate! Just don't go eating that whole family sized bar of chocolate every single night, or replacing your varied, healthy meals with too many giant size pizzas.

So what to do if you do pig out once in a while? Well don't worry too much either. We all have holidays where we camp out at the buffet breakfast until dinnertime, or have that birthday meal at a restaurant or times when we are tired and just want to be lazy and put our feet up with a snack. It doesn't matter. If it's only a day or two, then eat healthily for the rest of the week or pump up your exercise regime a bit to burn off the extra calories. It's no big deal. If it's longer, then do the same for a longer period. Healthy living and having a healthy diet is a long term, lifelong goal. It is a way of life, not a short term fix to do for a week or two before your holiday so you can hide your beer gut or fit into that bikini. That's not how it works.

What you need to develop is a healthy attitude to food. Food is wonderful, I love it! I love cooking it, eating it, sharing it with friends and family even; unless it is a big Hawaiian pizza, then woe betide anyone who goes near the last slice! Food is there to be enjoyed, not be scared of, not to deny yourself of it while you starve yourself on the latest fad diet. The trick is to ensure that the bulk of your diet is healthy, and everything else is taken in moderation.

Hydration, how much is enough?

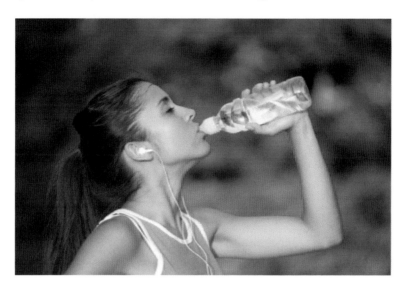

As most of you will know, we are mostly made up of water. Water keeps us alive, it supports metabolic reactions within the body, is the main component in our blood and helps carry various nutrients and compounds to where they need to be, as well as helping to get rid of all the waste products our body makes through urine via the kidneys. It helps us regulate our body temperature through sweat. Water is essential for our survival.

So it would be logical to assume that staying hydrated, and keeping the body topped up with water is essential to our health, and you would be right in doing so. Keeping our body's water balance correct and regulated is essential for our bodies to function. We lose water and fluid in a variety of ways, urination and sweat for example, so keeping that balance correct by drinking enough fluid is important.

> Myth buster! I need to drink 2 litres of water a day. This is a little bit of a myth based on misunderstanding. You have to drink at least 2

litres of fluid, it doesn't have to be just water, tea
or juice works just as well.

Current guidelines suggest that the average male needs to consume 2 litres of fluid per day, and women should take in 1.6 litres a day. It doesn't really matter if you drink more than that, in fact the more the better, because a healthy human body is fantastic at regulating itself and will have no problem getting rid of any excess fluid. It is important however that you do not drink less than this amount, as you will run the risk of dehydration and a variety of health problems that come with that. It is important to note though, that these guidelines are only a minimum, and should be increased if you live an active lifestyle or do a lot of exercise, or if you are in a hot or humid environment. Basically, if you are sweating a lot, then you need to drink a lot more water to make up for that weight loss.

Staying hydrated is essential in exercise. Basically the more you work out and the warmer you get, the more you sweat to cool yourself down, and the greater the need is to replace that fluid. Without water, your muscles will tire and you will become fatigued much more easily, and being dehydrated can even reduce your effectiveness by up to 30%. You may not even feel thirsty, but trust me, it will be having a detrimental effect. The best rule of thumb is to follow the old adage, drink before, keep drinking during, and drink plenty after exercise too.

Dehydration can be very dangerous, and even fatal over a sustained period. Over an extended period it can have negative health effects, but in the short term it can give you headaches, make you feel lethargic, increase the physical strain on your heart and have a detrimental effect on your ability to function. This effect is even more pronounced during exercise or in hot and humid conditions.

An easy way to measure if you are getting enough fluid or not is to check the colour of your urine. I know, not exactly a pleasant subject, but it works, trust me. If your urine is clear or very light straw coloured, then great. If it is really dark yellow or even brown coloured, then you are not getting enough fluid and need to drink a lot more.

However, what you drink can be just as important as how much. The common belief is that you must drink 2 to 3 litres of water a day. I hear this said so often and it is only half true. Yes, water is perhaps one of the best forms of fluid, but it isn't the only one. The fact is you must drink at least 1.6 to 2 litres of fluid per day. Not water, fluid. Fluid means water, juice, tea, any type of drink really. So if you are an otherwise healthy adult male, and only have 1 litre of water a day, but you are getting at least another litre of fluid from tea and diluted juice, then that can be fine too. You do have to be aware however that certain drinks are better than others, and some may have the exact opposite effect that you want to achieve.

Water is perhaps the best and most simplest forms of fluids out there. You simply can't beat it. But I don't know anyone who can or would even want to exist on water alone! Drinking a lot of it is great, but sooner or later you will want something different, and diluted fruit juice is just as good. It is after all still mostly water, it just tastes a bit better! Soft drinks that are high in sugar are absolutely fine in moderation, but taken in excess without any balance in terms of other drinks or exercise, then the high sugar content can bring with it an increased chance of obesity. Also, drinks such as coffee, some soft drinks and even some tea to a small extent contain caffeine too which has a small dehydrating effect on your body, which again is okay in small amounts, but must be countered by ensuring your overall fluid intake is adequate. Alcohol on the other hand, cannot be counted toward your total fluid intake at all because it dehydrates the body to the extent that it works as a diuretic. This means you will lose more fluid through urine than you will put in, and probably means you won't be all that popular at work if you make it a primary source of your fluid intake!

Sports drinks have become increasingly popular amongst athletes and gym goers in recent years, and whilst most are fine you do need to be aware of what is in them as they can make a difference to your workout and health. Those that are extremely high in sugar content are designed to rapidly replace fluids and glucose in your bloodstream to provide you with a quick and short burst of energy. These are great in moderation during prolonged exercise, however should only be used in moderation and certainly not consumed to excess without exercising. Too many of these drinks, especially the high energy drinks that contain large amounts of caffeine too can lead to increased strain on the heart and cause cardiovascular problems, so just be careful. Other sports drinks are designed to replace a range of other things dependent on the specific drink like electrolytes, carbohydrates, potassium and other nutrients that are lost during exercise and are a great way of staying hydrated and can even help your performance whilst exercising for longer periods of time.

If a healthy diet is this easy, then why have all my diets failed?

I hope that I have gotten my point over to you by now that the term 'diet' should no longer mean one of those fad regimes that you follow for a week or two before that holiday in the sun because you don't want to look a state in the holiday snaps. The term should be used to describe your overall healthy, balanced food and drink intake over a long, sustained period of time, hopefully your lifetime.

People often 'fail' diets because they don't think of it in that way, they think of it as something they should do to fit into that dress or lose that gut and go out and try and find a quick fix solution. These always fail sooner or later because they forced you to follow some strict regime or plan that didn't feel natural, so you gave up and went back to your old ways after that chocolate bar in the fridge forced itself into your mouth at gunpoint, honest guv'nor! If by chance you do manage to stick the regime out for a couple of weeks or so, then you may very well have lost a few pounds or more depending on how much the specific fad diet demands you starve yourself, but then you go and put it straight back on the second you came off it and went back to your old ways. This is because it isn't true, healthy weight loss. More often than not this 'weight' loss is down to muscle and fluid, not body fat at all, so you aren't losing the body fat in a healthy way. Often the reverse is true and you store extra body fat because your body has gone into starvation mode. Yes, your body is like a stroppy teenager, feed it, or it will punish you.

Don't view this advice as 'a diet'. View it as a way to completely overhaul your eating habits and have a healthy balanced diet for the rest of your life that will allow you to not only lose weight healthily, but also get all the nutrients your body needs, and allow you to enjoy food the way it is supposed to be! Now that sounds like a wonder diet!

Part 3 - Exercise.

Exercise conjures up almost as much anxiety in some people as the word diet does. It is something alien, something to be feared. How many of you have got an expensive membership to a gym that you never use but still burns a hole in your bank account every month? How many of you have actually made it over the threshold of a gym's doorway only to be intimidated by all the strange machinery and buff people in lycra admiring their muscles? How many have stared in awe and envy at all those people stretching into poses you thought were reserved for the Kama Sutra or sprinting a marathon on the treadmill whilst happily chatting away to their mate on the next one? I can imagine most people felt like that the first time they stepped through the gym doorway, but it is absolutely unnecessary.

First of all if you do decide to use a gym, then they can be great places to work out and not scary at all. You will not make a show of yourself when you fall flat on the treadmill, and no one will laugh at you or judge you. Even when you can't quite do as much as the bloke you have just seen running who you swear you saw in the Olympics. It isn't like that at all. Gyms are full of people just like you, just trying to improve themselves with exercise. Besides, gyms are full of people who can offer you help and advice when you need it too, there are quite often instructors around who are more than happy to help, as well as personal trainers if you need or want them. Not that I'm saying they are necessary of course. Many gyms also have various classes, which many people enjoy because it is different, you get the companionship of group work instead of just listening to your mp3 player, and many can give you a good cardio workout.

But bear in mind too that if you really don't like gyms or don't want to pay the monthly fees, they are not the only way to get fit, there are dozens of ways to exercise outside of them too. Play a sport, go swimming, run outdoors or exercise at home. It doesn't really matter, as long as you do some form of exercise.

There are so many different types of exercise it would be impossible for me to go too in depth with each one in this book, there are entire books devoted just to one specific type over another! Instead, I will give you a brief overview of the primary types of exercise you should be doing. I will give you the basic knowledge you need to train correctly and show you a few basics that you will need to know, and I will leave it up to you to tailor that knowledge into an exercise regime that suits your individual personality and needs. First though, we need to tackle the barriers to training, and the things you will need to know before you even start exercising.

Excuses, excuses, excuses!

I constantly hear people say that they don't need to exercise because they have this job or that job and spend all day on their feet. Men in particular who have active, physical jobs such as builders constantly use this as an excuse not to exercise, but is it true? Well this is partially true, it all depends on what your goals are.

It is true that daily activity in and of itself can burn calories. Of course it does, you are using up energy, right? And it is obvious that a job such as a manual labourer will require more physical energy than a secretary for example. So those people in very active jobs, or those who walking to the shops, carry home the shopping or do a lot of housework daily will expend energy in doing those tasks, and will therefore burn up some calories. It depends how vigorously you do the hoovering I suppose. So yes, if you control your calorie intake, and burn off more than you consume by doing a lot of activity, you will technically lose a little weight.

However, the calories burnt off with simple activities such as housework are not all that much compared to true exercise, and your daily activities in general will not in any way make you fitter, stronger or healthier. Unless you are extremely unfit and live an extremely sedentary lifestyle to begin with, all of these daily activities are simply considered as a normal part of life and daily energy expenditure, and your daily calorie intake already takes this into account. Burning off a few calories whilst rushing around the office is in no way going to get your cardiovascular fitness up. You just can't replace exercise with the excuse that you do a lot of housework or you have a busy, active job. So to make that very clear, everyday activities such as housework do not count in any way toward your daily aerobic or anaerobic exercise goals. So sorry everyone, stop making excuses and get your backsides off the couch! Even if your job is fairly physical, unless your day job is a famous sports star or Olympic athlete, you will still need to do some exercise during the week to maintain your cardiovascular fitness, strength and overall health. If you want to burn off more calories to lose a significant amount of weight over time, or your goals include getting fit or toning up too, then I'm afraid you will have to add exercise to your routine, there is no way around it.

> Myth buster! I don't have time to exercise! Of course you do. Ask yourself honestly how much time you spend slobbing in front of the TV or sitting updating your Facebook status! Start out with just a few hours per week, that is just 3 or 4 hours out of 168! Not much is it?

One of the most common excuses I hear on an almost daily basis is that 'I don't have time to exercise'. Men and women are just as bad as each other, but to use one of you as an example I hear all the time from many women about their martyrdom status, how they have everything in the world to do and no time to do it in, the kids to look after plus the daily grind of work all in the same day, so how dare anyone suggest that they exercise on top of that? Sorry ladies, that cuts you no slack here. It is an excuse just like any other, nothing more, nothing less, and the sooner you admit that the sooner you can get over it and start getting fitter and healthier.

If you are not used to exercise or much physical activity at all, you will benefit a lot from small starts. There are easy ways to incorporate exercise into your daily routine. It doesn't have to just be setting aside time to go to the gym, although if you want to do that then great. You don't even have to do all the exercise at once to begin with, split that half an hour daily recommendation up into three 10 minute mini workouts throughout the day instead. Why not have a fast walk to school with the kids so that you are all slightly out of breath, that helps the kids too! Take the kids swimming on a Sunday instead of sticking a DVD on? If you work really long days, and a lot of people do, then fit it around your work, I'm sure you have at least a couple of days a week off don't you? If you are one of those who does 14 hour days 6 or 7 days a week then quite frankly you need to cut back on your work or change your job. You are working too many hours and it is not healthy. I'm a staff nurse, and I work some off the longest, most stressful and most antisocial shifts that are available in the workplace, and I can still manage to fit my workouts and training around it on my days off. So if I can manage it, there is no reason anyone else can't. Just stop using all of these things as an excuse!

How much do I need to exercise?

The current guidelines for adults aged 19 - 64 are 2 and a half hours each week of moderate cardiovascular exercise, and that includes anything that gets your heart rate up a bit and you out of breath and a little sweaty, plus strength training on all major muscle groups twice a week. Those aged 18 or under should be doing an hour each and every day.

It is suggested that by fulfilling this minimum standard of exercise (and eating a healthy diet and maintaining a healthy body fat level too), you are cutting your risk of cardiovascular disease, heart disease, stroke and type 2 diabetes by more than half. The more you do, the better these odds get, and the more health problems you are likely to avoid.

Most people don't get anywhere near this level of exercise, and assume that they will have to do a lot to even achieve it. That is simply not the case. Remember, this is only a minimum recommendation, and what is considered moderate cardiovascular exercise really isn't difficult to incorporate into your life. Moderate intensity exercise can be something as simple as walking fast or cutting the grass, if you do it to the extent where you feel slightly out of breath and break into a mild sweat. Riding a bike or playing a sport such as tennis or football for half an hour will achieve this very easily. So half an hour a day for 5 days a week, and you have achieved that goal. Even sex is something that can be incorporated into your fitness regime! I know it isn't something that they offer classes in down at that posh gym, but think about it, can you think of any greater motivator to get you out of breath and sweating a little bit? It all helps.

Remember though that these guidelines are only a minimum recommended amount, and I would personally suggest using this as a starting point and gradually increasing it. If you are not used to exercise at all, then yes you will get a lot of benefit out of these minimum recommendations, but eventually you will hit a wall and find that half an hour of moderate exercise a day is not enough.

The amount of exercise you do is completely down to you as an individual and what your current fitness levels and your individual goals are. If your normal routine is very sedentary and your end goal is to lose a lot of body fat and be able to run a marathon in a year's time, then this minimum amount will not even come close. You will need to increase it month by month as you get fitter and healthier.

Balance in all things, Grasshopper!

To live a truly healthy lifestyle, balance in exercise is just as important as balance in your diet, and no I don't mean trying to do the crane stance on a wooden plank Daniel san style. I am talking about incorporating a full fitness regime into your life so that you can be fit and healthy and have great cardio fitness, but you can also have a strong and flexible body too. Your whole body is like a machine, and every single part needs to be functioning well if you are to maintain optimum health. There is no point in exercising one area to an extreme if you neglect other areas, as this can lead to problems too.

We have all seen those blokes down the gym who have very little clue about what they are doing, often grunting like Neanderthals about what supplement they are taking and who are only interested in buffing up their arms and chests so spend endless hours doing bicep curls and bench presses and nothing else, then end up looking like Gorillas with ridiculously out of proportion muscles in those areas but tiny waists and skinny legs. They look absolutely ridiculous preening themselves in front of the fancy full length mirrors. Don't worry about laughing at them, they have no cardio fitness so will never be able to catch you. You may have even seen that person on the treadmill who has great cardiovascular fitness because all they ever do is run, run, run, but looks ill because they have so little body fat and poor posture. They will end up with a lot of musculoskeletal problems later in life because the wear and tear will build up from years of high impact exercising and poor posture, and they don't have the muscle strength, tone or flexibility to be able to counter all the problems. Focusing largely on a particular exercise or sport is absolutely fine, as long as you mix your training up and get a range of benefits from a variety of other exercises too.

To achieve a perfectly balanced, healthy exercise regime, you need to do a little bit of everything. You need to keep your cardiovascular fitness up of course, that is essential, but you also need to improve your posture and flexibility, and you will need to strengthen and tone all of your major muscle groups, not just one or two.

So for example if all or most of your fitness regime is devoted to running or jogging and you do this 5 times a week, then simply cut that down to 3 or 4 and go swimming once a week and devote one session to flexibility and strength training too. Every once in a while give the running a miss for an extra session and go on the rowing machine or the cross trainer too. The same is true if you play a lot of sports, whatever your sport is, devote one session a week to pure cardio training, and another on specific strength workouts, and your performance will improve immeasurably. To be honest the actual mix is unimportant, and will largely depend on your individual interests and training goals, as long as you get at least the minimum amount of exercise a week and get a mixture of exercise types.

Be realistic and set realistic goals.

First of all you need to determine exactly what stage of health you are at now, and you have to be absolutely and completely honest with yourself here. There is no point in deluding yourself that you can secretly outrun everyone who did that marathon a short while back if you wanted to, or your call up for the Olympic try outs will come any day now if you have never stepped foot into a gym before. Be realistic.

Goal setting is essential in exercise, especially when you are just starting out. And it really doesn't matter whether the goal is to lose weight, run a marathon, participate in a sport or become a Herculean god, start small and build up to it.

It is absolutely fine to have general goals like those above as your ultimate aim, but the secret is to have smaller, measurable goalposts that you can hit along the way. It is important to be realistic here, as you will only be setting yourself up to fail if you set the bar too high to begin with. Do you want to run a marathon? Well start off by seeing if you can jog for 10 minutes, and make that your goal if you can't. Then build that up to half an hour, then an hour, and increase the speed at which you run each time. That way you can measure your progress. You can tell you are getting fitter and faster stage by stage, step by step, and I cannot stress enough the psychological benefits of achieving each small step on your motivation to continue.

Don't be afraid of changing your goals or your routine either. No one can predict the future and you may find that you have hit a goal early and you feel you can push yourself more, or you may find that you can't quite lift that weight you wanted to after a few months. It doesn't matter, just adjust your goals and your training accordingly and you will get there.

Technique, technique, technique!

One of the most common sights at the gym, apart from people admiring themselves in the full length mirrors of course, is people who are using incorrect techniques when exercising, particularly in strength training such as lifting weights.

We seem to live in a world now where people want results instantly, they don't want to put in the time and effort that is required. They expect just to walk into a gym and see Adonis like results within a week. This just won't happen and it leads to some really poor practice. This ranges from the bloke who comes in and starts swinging the heaviest weight about, using momentum rather than technique in an effort to look all manly and in the vain belief he will suddenly look like a bodybuilder, or those who can't even finish their sets because they have picked the wrong weight to those who slump themselves over the treadmill, leaning on the cross bars as their legs move at walking pace. At best these people are just wasting their time (and getting in everyone else's way as they hog equipment at busy times), at worst they can do themselves some serious injury.

I cannot stress enough the importance of correct technique and form. Exercising is important, but doing it right is too! All those little diagrams on the weight machines at the gym are not just for show, they are there to instruct you on the exact form you should use when performing the exercise. When exercising incorrectly, you will not only not achieve the results you want, or at the very least not achieve them as quickly or efficiently, but more often than not you will put unnecessary stress on your body which can lead to injury.

The most common injuries when performing any kind of strength training are to the back, the joints, and the muscles themselves. The lower back in particular is susceptible to injury, and muscles and joints too are commonly hurt when picking up too heavy a weight or training incorrectly. One thing I see almost every time I am in the gym is a bloke picking up the heaviest weight he can and swinging it upwards instead of doing a proper bicep curl. Using too much weight is a common mistake, and will have more negative effects than positive ones. You should train for your size and strength, not to show off or massage your ego. Pick a weight that allows you to complete the correct number of sets and reps that you need to accomplish your goals. If you aren't getting anywhere near that number, get a lighter weight. Secondly, in a bicep curl is an isolation exercise, and the only muscle that should be used is the bicep itself. By swinging the weight instead of lifting it in a controlled manner, then the effectiveness of the exercise is greatly reduced as you will not be isolating the muscle you want to train.

The best advice I can give you in a book such as this is basically to seek advice from a qualified trainer, who can show you the correct technique for individual exercises personally. Remember, these are the experts and are fully qualified to give you advice, so use them! Don't be shy, just ask! A book such as this with diagrams in it can only go so far, but I will try to give you a few basic pointers to start you off.

There are three basic rules to exercising safely, particularly if you are using weights or weighted machines or any type of flexibility exercise.

1. Use the correct weight for you as an individual. Don't try and lift too much because that is what you have seen others do. You'll hurt yourself unless you build up to that.

2. Use slow, controlled techniques that isolate the muscle or muscles you want to train for any given exercise. Rushed, half hearted or wild swinging techniques will not get you anywhere.

3. Breath. Just breath. Don't hold your breath, breath irregularly or make strange and unnecessary grunting or blowing sounds when you lift weights. That just makes you look like a fool and creeps out everyone around you. Breathing properly, deeply and naturally will help you control your technique and will give you the strength you need to train with weights by allowing blood to flow more freely, without putting undue pressure on your heart and lungs.

So please, apart from sticking to these basic common sense rules, just learn the proper techniques before embarking on any type of exercise regime. It will help you remain injury free, and it will get you better gains in the long term as you progress toward a healthy, strong body slowly and steadily.

Types of exercise.

There are essentially three primary types of exercise. Flexibility exercises, aerobic exercises or cardio, and anaerobic exercises or strength training. These three types between them cover the human bodies holistic fitness needs, including the numerous categories of physical skills that the human body requires to function, cardiovascular and respiratory endurance, strength, flexibility, stamina, agility, power and balance.

What this means in reality is quite simple, to live a healthy, balanced lifestyle, you need to be strong, you need to be flexible and you need to be fit. There is no point in being an ultra strong body builder if you can't climb a set of stairs without wheezing, or being able to complete a marathon easily if your body isn't flexible or has poor posture. Whilst many of us will have a natural tendency to do more of what we enjoy most or more of what exercise best meets our fitness goals, and this is fine to some extent, it is a good idea to get a general balance and train in all different aspects of fitness.

Flexibility exercises and stretching.

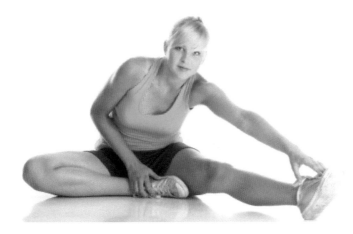

Flexibility is an essential function of the human body, and it is perhaps the single most overlooked aspect of any exercise programme. At best it is often relegated to a quick stretch before or after exercising, but this is a huge mistake. Flexibility can be a type of exercise regime in and of itself.

Flexibility is simply the range of movement available to the human body. Although there are slight differences in gender and between individuals, every single joint, limb and muscle has a range of movement that you should be able to achieve with a healthy body, and it is important for your mobility, health and exercise effectiveness. Poor flexibility can leave you much more prone to injury and long term health problems such as osteoarthritis and poor posture.

Stretching is a form of flexibility exercise that most people will be familiar with. Stretching utilises specific movements and poses to stretch the muscles elasticity, increase muscle tone, align the skeleton, increase flexibility and range of motion, and improve balance. Stretching is absolutely essential to living a healthy, active lifestyle, and being flexible can improve your quality of life, and your exercise effectiveness.

Like any form of exercise however, flexibility exercises can be confusing, especially for a beginner. There are a lot of different types, different styles, classes, and a lot of conflicting advice on when and where to actually do it. Hopefully, the next few pages will give you an understanding of the basics and let you determine what type of flexibility exercise is best for you.

Types of stretching.

Many of you will be familiar with stretching in some form or another, even if it is just knowing that is what you do first thing after you wake up! But many others will be aware of stretching as something to do before a workout, and they would be absolutely right. It is. The right type of stretching is important before and after exercise, but it is also important not to view stretching as just something to do at the start or end of a workout, but as a whole workout in and of itself. Stretching is relatively easy to incorporate it into your regime, of course still stretch before and after exercising, but why not devote a whole workout just to flexibility exercises? Or just have half an hour of stretching in the morning before you go to work?

The best thing about stretching is that it is relatively effort free and is an exercise system that is available to everyone, of all ages and abilities. Flexibility exercises and classes are perfect for the elderly, pregnant women and provided that you put the effort in and dedicate specific sessions to flexibility then you will feel the benefits to your fitness levels, your general health and well being, make you feel much more relaxed and less stressed, reduce the risk of injury both in and out of training and will hold off a lot of health problems for the future.

There are several different types of stretching and are either static (which involves no motion) or dynamic (which does require motion), and have a variety of exercises to facilitate each one. The different types of stretching are ballistic, dynamic, static, isometric, active and passive, and proprioceptive neuromuscular facilitation (PNF).

Ballistic stretching.

Ballistic stretching uses momentum, or bouncing, and puts the muscle into an extended range of motion, essentially trying to use momentum to force your limb or muscle to go further than it wants to. Bouncing up and down to touch your toes or swinging your leg or knee up repeatedly is an example of this type of stretch. I see people do it all the time in the gym and it really makes me cringe as unless you are training for a specific sport such as martial arts and absolutely know what you are doing in terms of correct technique, it is absolutely counter to what you should really be doing when stretching. What you should be doing is moving into each position slowly and gradually. Those who participate in sports which require a lot of jumping or explosive movements such as Karate often use this type of stretching, but evidence has shown it has little use beyond this specific type of activity and can often lead to injury if not done very carefully. So the next time you see guys on the football field jumping up and down, bouncing down to touch their toes or swinging their legs about, don't be tempted to copy them.

Dynamic stretching.

This is perhaps the type of stretch that most people find most beneficial and is perfect to use as a warm up before a workout or as a whole workout on its own. It involves slow and steady movements that gradually increase flexibility, reach and range of movement. Unlike ballistic stretching which involves fast, jerking momentum, dynamic stretching is slow and controlled. Yoga and Tai Chi embody this type of movement perfectly. Your limb should only go to the limits of your own range of motion, not beyond.

Dynamic stretches loosen up the muscles and increases your heart rate, temperature and blood flow, which makes it a perfect stretch to do before exercising. The walking lunge is an excellent example of a dynamic stretch, and yes, you may feel like a complete fool the first few times you do them (to be honest that never completely goes away), but you care less about how you look over time when you realise the benefits it has on your training. Leg lifts and walking bum kicks are also great examples. Have you ever been to a class, or can you remember those long forgotten PE classes in school where the instructor shouted at you to hit your bum with your heels as you jogged? Well that's dynamic stretching.

Active stretches.

These are those used a lot in martial arts, tai chi and yoga too. They are where your body assumes a stance or position and holds it there using only the strength of the muscles and balance. Imagine a Karate black belt bringing his leg up into a high kick position and then holding it there for a period of time.

Passive stretching.

This is when your body assumes a particular position to stretch a muscle, joint or tendon, but you use the assistance of something else to hold it there instead of your own muscle or balance. Imagine the same Karate black belt as before, but this time he has a partner or a piece of furniture to hold his leg in place and stretch his muscles. Passive stretching is often best used to cool down after a workout, as it is great at reducing lactic acid and muscle fatigue.

Static stretching.

Static stretching is very similar to passive stretching in a lot of ways, so much so that many people get the two confused. Like passive stretching, you hold or maintain a stretching position at the farthest point of your range of motion, but it is done from a still, or static position. The neck stretch where you may have seen people rolling their head slowly from side to side, dropping their ears toward their shoulders, is an example of this type of stretching. This type of stretching can be great for improving flexibility, but can be detrimental if you use it before a workout, especially a sustained cardio workout.

Isometric stretching.

This is perhaps one of the most effective ways to develop static - passive flexibility and uses passive stretching as a base from which to get greater flexibility gains. If you get into a passive stretch position, let's say the splits for example, then tense those muscles against the floor (or wall or partner, whichever is providing the resistance) for 15 seconds, then relax for 15 seconds and repeat. This works particularly well because basically, it brings much more of the fibres from the muscles being stretched into play by using the resting fibres as well as the stretched ones.

Proprioceptive neuromuscular facilitation (PNF) stretching.

Okay, this is a bit of a ridiculous name and not one that you need to worry about unless you get quite heavily into the technical side of fitness or become a health or fitness professional. Basically, it isn't really a technique in its own right, but combines passive stretching and isometric stretching. This method is used a lot by physiotherapists, and tries to take advantage of the elasticity of the muscle immediately after an initial isometric stretch by using a passive stretch and trying to stretch the muscle or limb beyond its initial maximum stretching capacity.

So which type of stretching is best for me?

Well to be honest, no one can really agree on that. Different sources will tell you different things. It really depends on what your individual goals are, what part of your session (warm up or cool down) you are performing or even what exercise you are doing. If you want to become a long distance runner for example, then dynamic stretching will be great for you as a warm up, and static stretches will help at the end of your run as you cool down. If you want to incorporate specific stretching workouts into your normal routine though, then I would personally argue a mixture of active and passive stretching would be a great way to go.

Whichever type of stretching you do, I would seriously recommend trying to do as much as you can as often as you can. If you can do half an hour daily on top of your other exercise, then that is ideal! Basically the more flexible you are, the better.

But before you do anything else, remember at all times, be safe. If anything hurts, stop! If you are unsure of exactly how to do something, ask an instructor! These are only basic tips, and you may need someone at first just to tell you if your technique or posture is right.

Stretching as a warm up.

During a warm up, you are essentially preparing your body for the stresses and strains you will put it through during exercise. You want your heart rate a little up, your blood flowing and your muscles relaxed and supple. To do that, you will need to stretch. Remember though that stretching is not a warm up on its own. It is just part of a warm up, and not even the first part! To raise your pulse and get your blood flowing a little first, simply do any type of mild incremental cardio exercise. These can include rowing, jogging, skipping or anything like that. You only have to spend 5 minutes or so doing this, you aren't aiming to completely tire yourself out before your workout!

Once you have warmed up a little, flexibility and joint mobility are your next major concerns, and this is where stretching comes in. Take your joints through their range of movement. It is important to slowly work your way through your whole body, bit by bit with simple, easy movements. A good way is to start at the neck, then the shoulders, and slowly work your way down to your feet. Range of movement exercises include slow neck turns by turning your head from left to right, slow shoulder rolls, bending the arms and rotating the wrists. There is nothing particularly technical or difficult about these, but they will allow the synovial fluid to help lubricate your joints and prepare them for exercise.

Dynamic stretching is perhaps one of the best types of stretches to use whilst warming up for any exercise programme, because they keep the heart rate and blood flow up and they get our muscles prepared for use and promote joint mobility. These are some useful dynamic stretches you can perform, although there are many more, so ask a trainer at the gym and find which ones work best for you.

Lunges.

This is a great, versatile exercise that has quite a few variations to get slightly different results, both static and dynamic, and can be done empty handed, with light dumbbells or even a light barbell on your shoulders to make it harder. Beginners should keep it light and easy however. They are great for exercising almost every muscle in the lower body, including the core to some extent because the stance leaves your body off balance and your core has to compensate. This variation is the most basic lunge, to make it dynamic, walk forward as you lunge on each leg.

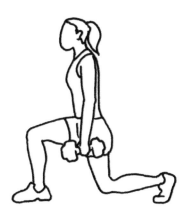

1. Stand with your feet shoulder width apart in a neutral stance.

2. Take a step forward in a wide stance.

3. Keeping your back straight and your head facing forward, bend your knees, your front leg should be bent at 90 degrees

and your back leg should be bent so that your knee is just above the floor.

4. Keep your weight evenly distributed as you come back up to a neutral stance and repeat on the opposite leg.

5. Try to do 10 lunges on each leg, you can work up to 15 and 20 lunges once you get used to them.

Squats.

These are excellent for strengthening and toning the thighs and backside. There are a number of variations on this, including assisted squats and barbell squats which we will come to later. This squat is the basic chair squat. It is not to be confused with the weightlifting stance. Beginners can actually place a chair behind them for safety, just in case they find they can't hold either the technique or their balance.

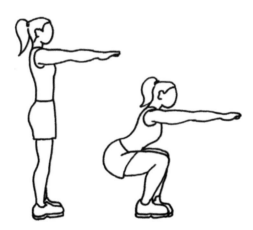

1. Stand with your feet shoulder width apart in a neutral stance.

2. Tense your abdominal muscles and slowly lower yourself down, bending at the knees and leaning forward slightly with

your upper body to maintain balance. imagine you are going to sit down in a chair.

3. How low you go is completely dependent on you, if you are not use to the exercise you might not be able to get too far, don't worry. If you can, try and aim for a 90 degree bend, as if you would be sitting in that invisible chair.

4. Hold the position from 5 to 30 seconds, the longer you can hold it, the greater the benefits, but do not push too far at first. When you are ready, slowly push back up with your legs and straighten your body. Repeat the movement 10 to 15 times.

Bum kick running.

This is technically a mild cardio exercise as well as a form of stretch, and will raise your heart rate a little as well as stretching your gluteal muscles, or your backside, as well as your hamstrings and quadriceps. There are a wide variety of ways to do this stretch as well as a wide variety of names. It can be done whilst jogging slowly around a small area, or jogging on the spot.

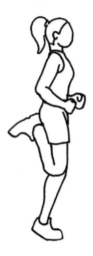

1. First of all simply start jogging normally, not too fast. Pay attention to the correct positioning of your arms and legs as you move, don't slouch.

2. As each foot hits the floor and you bring your other foot up, simply lift it behind you so that your heel touches your backside, not too hard, you aren't really aiming to kick yourself.

3. As that foot comes back down, bring the other foot up and repeat. Try and do 2 to 3 minutes to start with.

Side windmill lunge.

This is a good stretch for your core and will get your heart rate up too, especially if you keep the rate of lunges up.

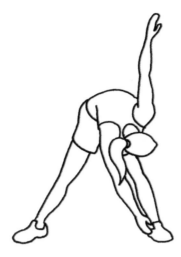

1. Stand with your feet wide apart and your arms directly out at your sides.

2. Bend one knee into a side lunge and swing your opposite arm down, touching your foot with the opposite hand.

3. Come back up to your starting position and immediately swing your other arm down and touch your opposite foot with your other hand. Repeat this for 30 seconds to a minute.

Stretching as a cool down.

Once you have performed your exercise specific cool down such as a slow jog or walk after a long moderate intensity run, then slow, static stretches are great for finishing your workout. They reduce the blood flow, hence slowing your pulse and reducing body temp, and relax muscles that have been used which helps stop any delayed onset muscle soreness, basically that ache you feel after lifting weights when you are not used to it.

Ideally you want to hold each stretch for at least 15 seconds, but holding each one for 30 - 45 seconds can not only help cool you down, but help increase muscle elasticity. There are a lot more, but some of the more common static stretches include:

Shoulder stretch.

As the name implies, this stretch targets your shoulders, more specifically the lateral deltoids, and is really important after any workout that incorporates shoulder movement that this stretch is done. It can help reduce the risk of injury such as impingement, and help increase the range of motion in the shoulder joint. Like a lot of stretches, it can easily be done either sat down or stood up.

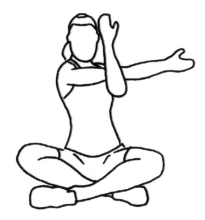

1. Stand with feet slightly wider than shoulder width, knees slightly bent.

2. Place your arm across your chest and use your other forearm to ease your arm across your chest until you feel a stretch in your shoulder.

3. Repeat with the other arm.

Side bend.

This is a great stretch for the core, the abdominal muscles and the side obliques in particular. But it can also stretch the shoulder and tricep muscles too to a smaller extent.

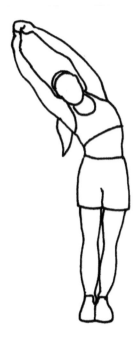

1. Stand with feet slightly wider than shoulder width, knees slightly bent.

2. Rest your hands on your hips and slowly bend to one side, letting your hand drop down your leg.

3. Slowly come back up to stand upright and repeat on the other side.

Triceps stretch.

This is a stretch for the back of your upper arm, or your tricep. Although you may feel a beneficial stretch to your shoulder too. It is an important stretch that can really help with the range of movement for your shoulder socket, and can be done either standing up, sitting down on a chair, medicine ball or floor. It doesn't really matter.

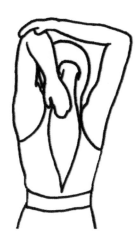

1. Sit or stand with your back straight.

2. Lift your arms straight above your head, palms forward, and bend one of your arms so that your thumb almost touches your head.

3. Now hold your elbow with the opposite hand and gently pull on your arm until you feel a stretch in your tricep. If you have difficulty reaching your elbow or have limited range of movement, then start off by holding your wrist and slowly work up to holding the elbow.

4. Repeat with the opposite arm.

Hamstring stretch.

Hamstrings are the muscles at the back of your thigh, and are an extremely important, if often overlooked, muscle to stretch, especially if you have been doing exercises such as running or playing sports. Stretching your hamstrings properly can help reduce injury after exercise, and even help promote flexibility and posture and reduce lower back pain. There are a variety of ways of doing this stretch, unlike other stretches though, standing or sitting involve different stretches altogether.

Sitting.

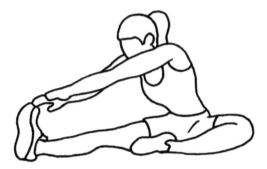

1. Sit on the ground with both legs directly out in front of you.

2. Bend one leg and place the bottom of your foot against your knee.

3. Bend forward slowly and in a relaxed manner, as if you are reaching for the foot furthest away from you.

4. Hold for 15 - 30 seconds. Repeat with the other leg.

Standing.

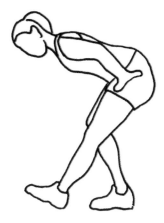

1. Stand up straight and step forward slightly so that the heel is in line with the toes of the opposite foot.

2. Bend the knee of your back leg slightly and lift the toes of your forward foot so that they are pointing upward and the foot is balanced on your heel.

3. At the same time, pull your abdominal muscles inward and lean your upper body forward. Rest your hands on the knee of your bent, rear leg for balance. You should feel the stretch in your forward leg which should be straight.

4. Repeat on the opposite leg.

Abductor stretch.

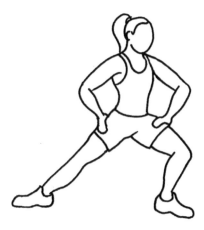

Your hip abductors are essential not just in sports and exercise, but to everyday life to. Without your abductors, you would have no mobility, it is as simple as that.

1. Stand with feet roughly two shoulder widths apart, knees slightly bent, as if you are sitting on a really fat horse.

2. Bend one leg and lower the body slightly to that side, keeping your back and other leg completely straight. You will feel the stretch in your hip abductor.

3. Repeat on the other side.

Seated groin stretch.

This stretch targets the abductors and the group of muscles on the inside of your thigh, the ones that extend from your pelvis to your knee. This is a really important stretch to help prevent injuries such as groin strain, but also to promote flexibility and mobility.

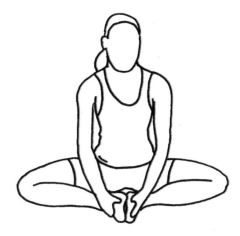

1. Sit down on the floor as if you were going to cross your leg, but put the soles of both of your feet together and pull them as close into you as is comfortable.

2. Keep your back straight and use your hands or elbows to slowly lower the knees to the ground.

3. Hold for 15 - 30 seconds. Remember to use slow, careful, deliberate movements, do not bounce your legs!

Stretching as a full on workout.

As I have said, stretching doesn't just have to be part of a warm up and cool down. Many people can benefit from devoting a session once in a while wholly to stretching and flexibility exercises.

Even if that session is coupled with specific flexibility workouts such as Pilates for example, or a balance session or even a light strength session, the increased time spent stretching can have tremendous stress relieving and relaxation properties, as well as giving you improved flexibility, body awareness and suppleness. Everyone can and should gain from this form of exercise, but the elderly, pregnant women and those recovering from injury or are not used to exercising at all can reap particular benefits.

There is nothing particularly difficult to learn, after a basic warm up to get your blood flowing, simply work through some of the dynamic stretches you would do normally, and then some slow, relaxing dynamic stretches and then a cool down. Do a lot more stretches than you would normally do and incorporate the whole body, even try out a few new ones. A good pointer is to extend the length of your stretches as you do them. If you normally maintain a stretch for 15 seconds say, try increasing each one to 30 seconds each, which will increase your flexibility in the long term.

Stretching with equipment.

Dynamic exercises are great for warming up, done in enough number and at a certain level of intensity, they can even be a mild workout in and of themselves for beginners. The few exercises given in previous pages are just a small sample, there are many more. One way in which to get a more intense warm up or add variety to your routine, is to use equipment. By stretching with equipment, you can not only increase the intensity of your stretches, but you can also develop mild strength gains too, dependent on the weight used. You can adjust the weight used dependent on your fitness levels and your training needs, using lighter weights for a warm up in one session, or increasing the weight and doing a wider variety of dynamic stretches if you want a light strength and flexibility workout. Medicine balls or kettlebells are really good for this purpose, and are often completely underused by many people.

Kettlebell exercises.

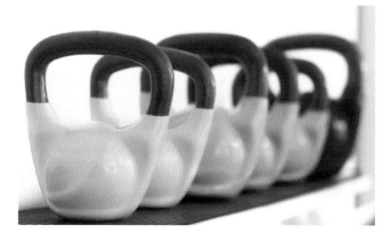

Kettlebells are weights in the shape of a ball with a handle protruding from the top. They have been used by the Russian special forces and infantry for a long time, and have recently become very popular in gyms and health clubs, being advertised as the ultimate and efficient strength training exercises. They are not like traditional free weights, because the techniques used in training with kettlebells often facilitate swinging movements or powerful ballistic movements, the exact opposite of what is often required in free weight training. That is why Kettlebells are great at advance levels for strength training, but they are also absolutely perfect for stretching too.

Some people argue that kettlebell training can replace other forms of exercise and be used as an effective all round routine on its own. Whilst I certainly would not recommend that, it is certain that kettlebells can be a great addition to a balanced routine.

I know that many people may be intimidated by these small balls of iron, that is easy to understand, they are strange pieces of equipment and the exercises are unfamiliar but with the right training in technique anyone can use kettlebells for a variety of exercise goals. For those of you who just want to tone up and get a good cardio workout with some dynamic training, then simply use one of the lighter weights. For those of you who want to turn up the intensity and build more muscle mass, then substitute the lighter weights for heavier ones. The techniques will be the same regardless.

Because of the ballistic nature of these exercises however, and because there is a lot of controlled swinging movements, there is a risk of injury for the beginner if the techniques are not performed right. For this reason, it is important that if you want to incorporate this training into your workouts, then you must seek advice from an instructor or trainer who is trained in their use.

Medicine ball exercises.

Medicine balls are a mainstay of most gyms and health centres, but are often reduced to simple abdominal exercises or even overlooked entirely by many people who may not know how to use them correctly. They are available in a wide variety of sizes and weights and are extremely simple to incorporate into your stretching and flexibility routine if you want to make your normal programme a little more challenging.

Choosing the right weight of ball is exactly the same as making sure that the free weight you use is correct for you. It can't be too light, or there is little point, but it can't be too heavy so that your technique is compromised and you cannot complete your normal sets. But once you have the correct weight, then you can construct a routine that develops your core, your balance and a wide range of muscle groups.

Just as with kettlebells however, it is important that you get the technique of each exercise just right so as to avoid injury, so it is a good idea to have an instructor show you what to do and make sure your technique is right before you start training on your own.

Yoga, Pilates and Tai Chi.

Many of you will have heard of Yoga, Pilates and Tai Chi. There has been a popularity explosion in recent years for these traditional forms of exercise, with many of the larger gym and fitness chains offering classes in at least one style, if not all three. It is very easy to see why, these exercise forms are low impact and very easy for people of all ages, shapes, sizes and fitness levels, and they all have a lot of health benefits. Despite their differences, they are all essentially based around flexibility and stretching exercise.

Let's get this straight, when I talk about these forms of exercise, I am not talking about the strange myriad of fad classes and DVDs that get churned out such as Yogacise, yin yang yoga or yoga dance or whatever mish mash of names they want to throw together. There have been a lot of classes in recent years that have blended yoga and Pilates together, because the two systems work very well together and quite frankly, people are always looking for the next new fad. It doesn't matter that the core exercises are all the same, people will shell out a lot of money for fancy classes with a name like yogilates, pilaga or extreme Pilates, despite the fact there is nothing new about them at all.

If that is what it takes to get you training then these classes don't really do any harm, as long as the instructor knows what they are doing (and are qualified and registered with their respective bodies such as the Register of Exercise Professionals, or REPS). Some people do enjoy the social aspect of classes like these and get a lot out of them, which is absolutely fine. But you really don't need to do any of these fad classes at all, or spend large amounts of money joining a fancy gym to get to them. The core aspects of Pilates and yoga are very, very simple and are easy to learn and incorporate into your own routine as you see fit.

It can however be easy to get confused about which class does what and what benefits are to be gained from doing any particular one over the other, because at a fundamental level there are a lot of similarities with the only obvious difference to a layperson being cultural. I'm talking here about the actual distinct art forms themselves, as they can be a fantastic addition to a flexibility exercise regime or a stretching programme. Even if you don't want to attend the classes themselves, or at least attend them all the time due to family or other commitments, it is very easy to pick up some of the basic techniques and incorporate them into your own regime. The easiest way to start this, is by having a little bit of knowledge about each one.

Yoga.

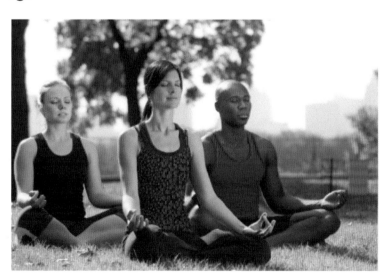

Yoga is more than just a form of exercise, for many it is a way of life. It is a bit of a general term encompassing a lot of different disciplines originating in India, and is a philosophy of living as well as a form of meditation and physical exercise. In modern exercise terms, it has come to mean a modern workout system where a variety of poses and stretches are utilised to boost physical and mental wellbeing, and increase flexibility and increase muscular strength, blood flow and posture alignment. You may have seen or heard of a wide variety of different types such as bikram yoga. Many are concerned with aspects such as spirituality or religion, which is absolutely fine if you want to discover Yoga on a deeper level, but hatha yoga is the one that is most popular in the West as it primarily focuses on health and physical exercise.

There have been a lot of clinical and scientific studies done on the health benefits of yoga, and whilst there have been varying results as to the extent of the benefit, the general consensus is that yoga is an excellent and safe form of low impact exercise. The physical benefits of yoga are generally quite obvious, improved flexibility, balance and posture, improved muscle tone and less risk of injury to say the least, but there has also been evidence to suggest that yoga can also be beneficial to arthritis, high blood pressure, back pain, depression and stress too.

Hatha yoga incorporates pranayama (breathing control), dhyana (meditation) and the different poses and stretches are broken up into groups, known as asanas, and are arranged depending on their benefit to your body. These physical postures involve every part of the body and are a great way to stretch, align and stimulate the muscles, skeleton and internal organs.

There are hundreds of asanas, each one designed to exercise a different part of your body. It is always best to start off at a class with a teacher who can show you the correct technique, even if you don't like classes and only attend a few to learn the basics, then that's fine, you can still practice the basic techniques at home or in your own space. If you want to do some of the more advanced poses, then joining a class and learning the techniques under proper guidance is pretty necessary. However, the basic ones can be learned quite easily and practiced in your own home or as part of your normal routine.

Getting started.

One of the best things about yoga is that you really don't need much at all to get started, it can be done anywhere, by anyone and without any special equipment. You don't need to get the latest in fitness fashion or fancy all white yoga clothes from that pretentious shop, all you need is loose, comfortable clothing and a clean, quiet and with enough room to spread out comfortably. Although not completely necessary, many people do find that a cheap, non slip mat and a foam block or a pillow to be an advantage, and if you want to continue yoga training over the long term then you will certainly find things more comfortable with them, but you don't have to worry about them to begin with. These poses are just a few of the basic poses that should give you a flavour of what yoga is all about. Guidance is given on how to perform the poses, but you may still need a teachers guidance to ensure your posture and technique is correct at first, particularly if you are a beginner.

Warm up and finishing poses.

Just as in any exercise, a thorough warm up and cool down is essential. Many beginners find that some of these restorative exercises bring great benefits in and of themselves, and many people do so just as part of a daily routine, as they are designed to open up and align your body, restore and rest your muscles and skeleton and can make you feel really relaxed. Meditation is often a part of these restorative exercises, and many beginners have found that it is extremely easy to drift off whilst doing these. Don't worry if you do, most people do exactly the same, myself included once or twice!

Corpse pose (Savasana).

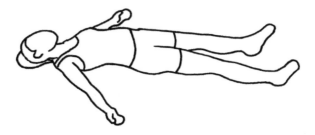

1. Lie down on your back with your arms relaxed at your sides, palms up, and your legs straight, feet hip width apart.

2. It is essential that your body is in a neutral position for this pose, so try and find a position where your lower spine is not flat on the floor, but is not arched either. Your stomach should be completely flat too. Some people find it useful to use a folded towel or a pillow under their spine at first until they get used to it. Your head should be positioned so that the base of the skull is away from your neck and in line with your spine. You may need an instructor at first just to make sure that you are getting the neutral position correct, but once you are used to it you will find it very natural to do.

3. Once in neutral position, try to stay in this pose for at least five minutes and concentrate on controlling your breathing

and softening and relaxing each and every one of your organs, starting at your brain and working down.

Childs pose (Balasana).

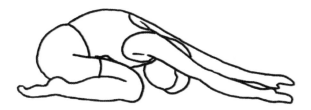

This is a very restful pose that stretches the thighs, hips, spine and shoulders. Many beginners find it easier to do with a foam block or folded towel under their knees for support.

1. Kneel on the floor, sitting on your heels with your ankles and feet together. Your knees should be hip width apart from each other.

2. Exhale slowly and lean forward, stretching your arms outward with your palms flat on the floor and your forehead not quite touching the ground.

3. You should feel a comfortable stretch along the length of your torso and along your spine.

4. Stay in this position from 30 seconds to a few minutes, whatever feels comfortable!

Standing poses.

Standing exercises are an essential part of yoga and not only improve your posture and your balance, but open up the hips and trains and stretches the legs, lower back and spine.

Mountain pose (Tadasana).

This is the basic standing form that most beginners will learn and is the basis of a lot of standing poses. This is an excellent pose to simply become aware of your entire body, bit by bit, and ensure that your posture and alignment are correct. Most beginners stand against a wall to help them at first, but it is a really good idea if you are practicing at home just to attend a class or two with an instructor who can ensure you are getting the posture correct.

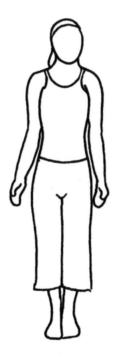

1. Stand up straight with your arms by your side and your palms out, and your feet together.

2. Your weight should be completely balanced on your feet, and you should be able to rock back and forth and side to side easily.

3. Align your spine to its neutral position and your head in line with your pelvis. Turn the upper thighs slightly inward, imagine your tailbone lengthening toward the floor and widen your collarbones.

Chair pose (Utkatasana).

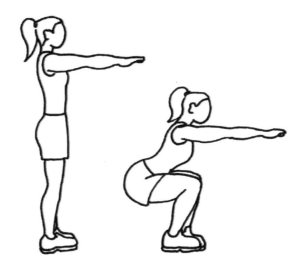

1. Start off in mountain pose.

2. Inhale slowly and raise your arms above your head, palms together.

3. Exhale and bend your knees as if you were sitting on an invisible chair.

4. Keep your legs together and your knees slightly over the feet. Your chest should be leaning forward slightly but your spine should still be in alignment as your tailbone is thrust out slightly too.

5. If you are a beginner or have mobility or joint problems, you may not be able to get down very low at first, that's okay it is

normal. Just keep doing it and your strength and mobility will quickly improve.

Downward facing dog (Ahdo Mukha Svanasana).

This is another classic pose and one that most people will be able to do with a bit of practice.

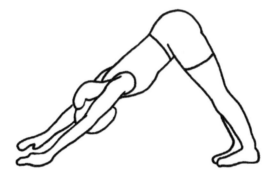

1. Kneel on the floor on all fours and hold your palms slightly out in front of you, spreading your fingers so that your hands have a wide base.

2. Exhale slowly and push your knees up from the floor, lifting your tailbone up to the ceiling.

3. Your feet should be flat on the floor and your knees should not be bent.

Seated poses.

Sitting poses allow you to attain the correct breathing and can help with relaxation and meditation.

Staff pose (Dandasana).

This is a very basic pose that requires the full alignment of your upper body. It is one of the very first that many beginners learn and is the basis of many other techniques.

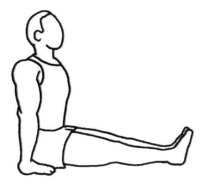

1. Sit on the floor with your back straight and your legs together and straight out in front of you.

2. Your spine should be in neutral position. Some beginners find it easier to sit against a wall for this, as it is easy to measure the neutral position. Your shoulder blades should be touching the wall, but your head and your lower spine should be away from it.

3. Press down your thighs into the ground and imagine your spine lengthening as you pull your groin toward your sacrum.

Bound ankle pose (Baddha Konasana).

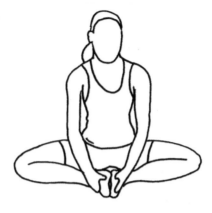

1. Sit on the floor in the staff pose with your spine in a neutral position and your legs out in front of you. Again, like in many seated poses, some beginners or elderly find that sitting on a foam block or a folded towel can help with this if they have restricted mobility, don't worry if you need to, it can take time get the flexibility needed just keep at it.

2. Exhale slowly and bend your knees so that your heels come toward your groin.

3. With the soles of the feet together, slowly lower your knees to the floor so you can feel a stretch in your inner thighs. This should be a smooth, relaxed movement, never bounce your knees or force them down. You can hold your feet with your hands, or your ankles if you cannot quite reach the feet yet, but don't pull them in further than is comfortable for you.

4. Stay in this pose for 1 to 5 minutes.

Lotus pose.

This is one of those fundamental yoga poses that people conjure up when they imagine yoga practitioners, but it can be quite difficult for beginners. This is one that should be done with an experienced teacher in a class.

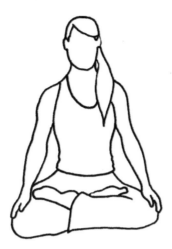

1. Sit on the floor in the staff pose with your spine in a neutral position and your legs out in front of you.

2. Bend your knees and use your hands to cross your legs so that the top of your left foot is resting against your right thigh and the top of your right foot is against your left thigh.

3. Lean back slightly so that your spine is stretched and you can feel the full range of movement in your hips.

4. If you find this comfortable and are sufficiently flexible, then you can gently press your thighs down with the sides of your feet.

5. Many people use this pose for meditation and place their hands in a 'mudra', which is a symbolic gesture said to bring about levels of consciousness in meditation. But you don't have to do this if you don't want to.

Core poses.

Cat pose (Marjaryasana).

This is great for aligning the spine and stretching the stomach muscles.

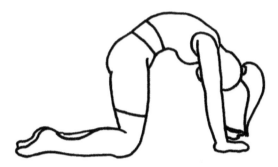

1. Start by leaning down on all fours, your palms should be shoulder length apart and facing the same direction, and the tops of your feet should be on the floor. Your knees shouldn't be too far apart either, try and get them in line with your hips.

2. Keep your head lifted so you are looking down to the floor but your head isn't hanging down.

3. With a slow exhalation, slowly arch your spine upward. The spine should be the only part of you that is moving.

4. Imagine each and every segment of the spine separating and stretching as you move, lower your head slightly at the same time.

5. As you inhale, slowly come back down to the starting position.

Cow pose (Bitilasana).

This is often done alongside the cat pose, one after the other, as they flow into each other really well. But you can do them separately if you want to.

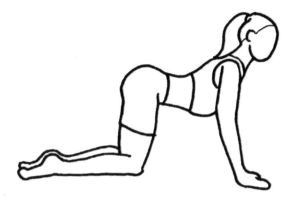

1. Start on your hands and knees in the same position as the cat pose, but this time instead of arching the back upwards, you are doing the exact opposite.

2. As you inhale, lower your belly and lower back toward the floor, and lift your chest and sacrum up toward the ceiling.

3. Lift your head so that you are looking directly forward.

4. Exhale and come back to the starting neutral position slowly.

Twisting poses.

These release the tension in your spine and stretches the shoulder muscles and joints. They are also great at training your side obliques.

Marichi's pose (Marichyasana).

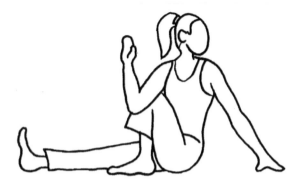

1. Sit in the staff pose with your back straight and your legs out in front of you.

2. Bend your right knee so that the bottom of your foot is on the floor and the heel is as close to your backside as you can get it.

3. Rotate your left leg very slightly inward and imagine your hips are weighted into the floor.

4. Exhale and very slowly rotate your torso and put your left arm straight against the outside of your right knee, effectively holding the technique in place. Use your right hand to balance yourself by holding it out to your right side behind you.

5. Keep your spine in alignment and twist that little bit further with each exhalation of your breath until you reach the point where you cannot comfortably twist any more.

6. Stay in this pose for 30 seconds to 1 minute, then slowly release the pose and repeat on the other side.

Bharadvaja's twist.

This is a great basic twist, women usually find this a little naturally easier than men.

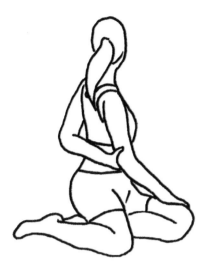

1. Sit on the floor and lean over slightly onto your right buttock, bringing your legs underneath you to the left. Your feet should be just by your left hip.

2. Slowly inhale and twist your torso to the right, slowly turning your head to the right at the same time. Keep your back straight and imagine it lengthening at the same time.

3. Hold your right knee with your left hand, and squeeze your shoulder blades together so you can hold your left arm with your right hand.

4. Stay in the position for 30 seconds to a minute, then slowly release, return to the starting position and then repeat on the other side.

Inverted and balanced poses.

These can be difficult for beginners, so don't worry if you can't get them straight away. They take time and practice to achieve. These are the poses that many people imagine when they think of yoga for the first time. Inverted and balanced poses use gravity as well as body strength to stretch your muscles, skeleton and joints. They are excellent for improving your balance, your overall muscle tone and strength as well as stamina.

Supported shoulder stand (Salamba Sarvangasana).

This is an inverted pose that is a little difficult to do at first, but can be achieved with a bit of practice and training. A lot of people, both beginners and otherwise, find that a folded towel or a foam block is really helpful and comfortable.

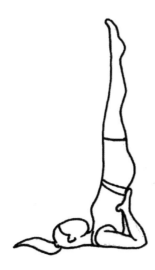

1. If you decide to use them, place the folded towels or the foam block on the floor. The aim is that your upper arms and the top of your spine will be on this when you execute the technique, so lay down on your back with your knees bent, your shoulders on the foam block and the back of your head on the floor. Place your arms at your sides so the backs of your upper arms are on the towels too.

2. Exhale slowly and push with both your feet and your arms so that your legs are drawn upward past your torso.

3. Keep this lift going by inhaling slowly and pushing your hips away from the floor and pointing your feet toward the ceiling. Your pelvis should be in line with your shoulders so that you are not off balance.

4. Place your hands on your lower back, but keep your elbows in the same position as they were when your arms were flat.

5. Try to keep this pose for 30 seconds. Once this feels comfortable you can extend this gradually until you can stay in the pose for a few minutes.

Crane pose (Bakasana).

This balancing pose requires a fair bit of strength from the arms, especially the triceps, and a good level of balance, so as with all of these poses do not worry if it takes time to get it right.

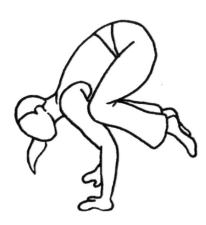

1. Squat down so that the soles of your feet and the palms of your hands are both touching the floor.

2. Lean forward slightly so that your weight is balanced through your arms.

3. Your elbows should be slightly bent and your knees out slightly further than your hips.

4. Press your knees into your armpits and your thighs close to your torso.

5. Lean forward even more and lift up onto the balls of your feet at the same time, then lift your feet off the ground.

6. Your triceps will be taking all of your weight now, make sure your spine stays rounded by consciously pushing your tailbone toward the floor and your feet into your backside as much as possible.

Tree pose (Vrksasana).

Another iconic yoga pose, this is a lot more difficult than it looks.

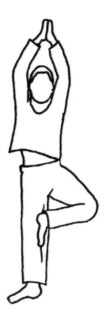

1. Start off in the basic tree pose so that your body is aligned and your mind restful.

2. Without changing position, shift all of your weight onto your right foot.

3. Slowly inhale, bend your knee and lift your foot up so that the sole is flat against your inner thigh with the toes pointing toward the floor. If your foot can only reach your inner knee, don't worry, that is fine for now.

4. Your body should be leaning very slightly so that the centre of your pelvis is over the foot on the ground. Lengthen your tailbone toward the floor and ensure your spine is in the neutral position.

5. Slowly lift your arms up above you and bring the palms of your hands together.

Backbends.

These are great for the back as well as the stomach, releasing tension in your lower back, hips and pelvic girdle. They also help improve the flexibility and posture of the spine.

Cobra or snake pose (Bhujangasana).

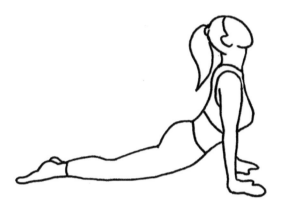

1. Lie down on your stomach and stretch your legs out, keep your ankles together and the tops of your feet on the floor.

2. Put your palms on the floor by your shoulders and press your feet and pubis into the floor.

3. Inhale slowly and lift your upper torso up, use your arms for support only, it isn't a push up.

4. Push your shoulder blades against the back and your chest outwards, so your lower back is arched. Don't overdo this arch, make sure it is comfortable and you are not straining your back.

5. Hold the position for 15 to 30 seconds before slowly coming down to a prone position again as you exhale.

Bridge pose (Setu Bandha Sarvangasana).

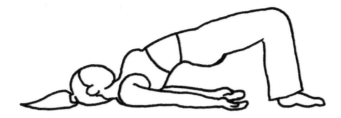

1. Lie down on the floor in a neutral position.

2. Slowly raise your knees until your feet are flat on the floor, as if you were going to do an abdominal crunch, but try and bring your feet as close to your hips as is comfortable for you.

3. Some beginners find it more comfortable to place a folded towel under their shoulders before attempting this.

4. When you are comfortable, exhale slowly and push your tailbone toward your pubis until your hips lift off the floor.

5. Stay in this position for 15 to 30 seconds before exhaling and slowly lowering your hips to the floor.

Pilates.

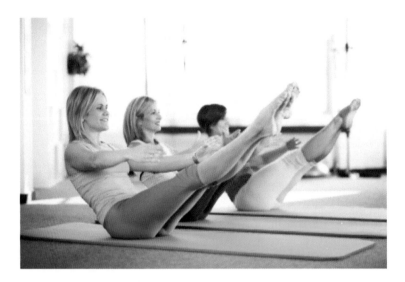

There is a lot of myth and confusion about Pilates, that it is a martial art, or a wonder cure for anything and everything from back pain to obesity. The truth is, it is not really any of these. Pilates is a Western exercise system that at its core has a lot of similarities to Yoga and other art forms, in that it uses exercises, breathing and other techniques to actively develop balance, flexibility, strength and alignment in the muscles and skeletal system of the body, but differs in the fact that it has no specific cultural or religious ideology.

Part of this confusion is down to the fact that there has been a lot of classes in recent years that have blended yoga and Pilates together, because the two systems work very well together and quite frankly, people are always looking for the next new fad. It doesn't matter that the core exercises are all the same, people will shell out a lot of money for fancy classes with a name like yogilates or pilaga or yoga dance or extreme Pilates, all with an excitable instructor.

If that is what it takes to get you training, then these classes don't really do any harm, as long as the instructor knows what they are doing. It is important to remember that there is no governing body that ensures that all Pilates classes follow the same structure, and there are a wide variety of styles and hybrids. Just find one that suits you and the way you train. Some people do enjoy the social aspect of classes like these, but you really don't need to do any of these fad classes at all. Like yoga, the core aspects of Pilates are very, very simple and are easy to learn and incorporate into your own routine as you see fit.

Pilates, like yoga does have a variety of health benefits for many people. It will make you more flexible and your muscles more toned and lean, this obviously will have benefits on general aches and pains, back pain in particular, and is a great way for the elderly or those recovering from an injury to do some training because it is a gentle, low impact exercise. It will not however make you lose weight or become slimmer, I don't care what that fancy poster on the gym wall says. A healthy diet and aerobic exercise is the best way to lose body fat, but what Pilates will do is strengthen and tone up your muscle underneath the fat, so that when you do lose some weight, your body looks more toned and buff.

Many people start up Pilates because they want to develop one specific area, usually the stomach because everyone wants that elusive six pack, but it stresses the importance of balance, stretching and strengthening the entire body.

Getting started.

The fundamental aspect of Pilates is an understanding and awareness of your body, the techniques are in effect simply tools to allow you to do this, whilst gaining coordination, strength, balance and flexibility. In order to change the way you move and the way your body works, then the body and mind must work together and bring about an unconscious control over how your movements become controlled and graceful. Two tenets central to this are breathing and core strength. You may hear them called by different names in the school or class you attend but they are essentially the same thing. Controlled breathing, synchronised with your body's movements, and the development of strong core muscles in your trunk are the basis of all movement.

There are two types of Pilates class, mat work and studio classes. Mat work might be the type that most people are familiar with as they are more widely available and are mostly performed on a simple mat, perhaps with occasional use of a resistance band. Studio classes on the other hand are not as common as they require a dedicated space and specific pieces of specialised equipment such as the Reformer or Ladder Barrel. These are essentially just machines to help you perform your Pilates techniques, but this is not something you have to worry about at first, if at all. If you want to go to a class as a beginner or even do some of the exercises at home, then all you need is a padded non slip mat for comfort, a small towel, an exercise band or a long scarf, and loose comfortable clothing. Most mat work classes will have spare mats and spare bands available if they use them.

Alignment.

This is a key principle in Pilates and fundamentally important to your basic health and posture. Alignment simply means the correct position of the body either standing, sitting or lying down, so that the skeleton, joints, ligaments and muscles are all exactly where they should be to reduce strain, wear and tear and pain. Many exercises and positions require that your body, particularly your spine and hips, are in the correct neutral, or natural position, others may require you to specifically move out of alignment to create stress for the exercise. An awareness of which is which is vital.

Many techniques in Pilates are used to promote and elongate the natural curve of the spine, similar to an elongated S shape, and develop the deep, postural muscles that allow for correct posture. Many of us have developed poor posture over many years, or even decades of sitting slumped on the sofa, carrying heavy bags on one shoulder or sat at the office desk hunched over a keyboard, not to mention the natural compressive effects of gravity, impacts and old age, so development of the natural shape of the spine can be beneficial to pretty much everybody at any time.

The natural or neutral position of the pelvis is important to the correct alignment of the spine, but is also important in and of itself. When the pelvis is neutral, the pubic and pelvic bones should not be tilted either backward or forward. The position of the head, neck and cervical spine are also important in correct alignment, and there are a variety of beginner positions to help you achieve this.

The neutral spine position.

Lie on your back with your feet flat on the floor and in line with your hips, as if you were about to do a sit up. Rest your arms at your side palms down. Keep in mind before you start the natural elongated S shape of the spine, you should not be trying to flatten your whole back against the floor. Relax and take slow, deep breaths. Try and find a position where your lower spine is not flat on the floor, but is not arched either.

Your stomach should be completely flat too. Some people find it useful to use a folded towel or a pillow under their spine at first until they get used to it.

Breathing.

Okay, I know everyone breathes, and I know we all know how to do it automatically, and that is true. So why need to learn how to do it differently? Well in Pilates, it is much more about learning to be aware of and control your breathing, similar in a lot of ways to systems such as Qigong in China which utilises controlled breathing to power the low impact movements. Breathing naturally incorporates a lot of muscles and does affect how we move. Take a conscious deep breath in, you should be able to feel the process of your lungs inflating and your ribcage expanding, your diaphragm will be lowering at the same time. Now slowly exhale, and you should be able to feel the air being pushed out from your lungs and your ribcage contract as your diaphragm rises.

Exercising these muscles can have great benefits if you are unfit and just started training, you are stopping smoking or you have a respiratory disease such as COPD, but it can also be a great way to focus and concentrate, essential for relaxation and meditation.

Core strength.

You may hear this aspect referred to as centring or centre strength or something similar dependent on your class and teacher, but whatever different disciplines call it, it is all about developing core stability, something that you will be familiar with from earlier chapters. The benefits of core stability should be self explanatory by now, but in Pilates, it also means being able to maintain full and complete control and awareness over all of your movements, so that your body can move to the best of its ability.

Mobility.

Mobility is essential in everday life, and is required to achieve even the most basic activities of daily living. Pilates not only stretches and improves the muscle tone in your body, which improves mobility in and of itself, but more importantly promotes the establishment of correct movement. The way we move is just as important as moving itself in many ways. Articulation of the spine is essential, and Pilates teaches you to do this very slowly, segment by segment, so that you can maximise the spines ability to bend forwards (spinal flexion), bend backwards (spinal extension), sideways (spinal lateral flexion), and twist (spinal rotation).

Hopefully understanding these basic tenets of Pilates will give you a grounding in the exercises and techniques used in the classes themselves. Even if you feel like the classes aren't for you, don't worry, these basic movements and positions will still have a lot of benefits. Just remember, Pilates is not a complete exercise system. It is an important part of a balanced lifestyle, but needs to be supplemented with cardiovascular and strength training too.

Tai Chi Chuan.

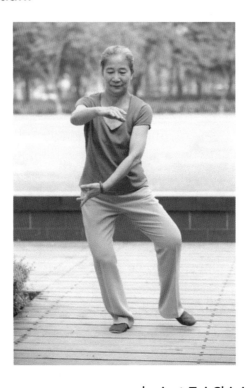

T'ai Chi Ch'uan, or more commonly, just Tai Chi, is an ancient Chinese martial art. That's right, unlike Pilates and yoga, Tai Chi is a martial art and does have a combat aspect to it. There are so many different styles of Tai Chi, most of them based on one of the traditional Chinese schools of Chen, Yang, Wu Hao, Wu and Sun in some way. Some styles are more traditional and cover the full curriculum from basic forms and pushing hands, right through to weapons training with the sword and fan, as they believe that the health benefits and the martial benefits of T'ai Chi Ch'uan go hand in hand, the Yin and the Yang. Others focus much more on the health benefits of Tai Chi, with meditation, hand forms and breathing exercises, known as Qigong. This is the most common form that is seen in many schools today, especially in the West, where Tai Chi is practiced as a simple form of health promoting exercise, with the martial art aspect left out for advanced practitioners only, and even then only those who want to train in that way. Many classes do not offer this option at all.

There are many different schools, or styles of Tai Chi, and all have slight differences in technique, but essentially Tai Chi is a system that uses slow, graceful movements to enter the postures and techniques that characterise each style. When done properly, it is very graceful and to the outsider looks almost like a dance. These techniques promote a lot of balance, flexibility and stretching within the skeleton and muscles, and will often flow very smoothly from one to the other.

The non combat, pure exercise form of Tai Chi has many health benefits similar to yoga and Pilates, as it too is a low impact form of gentle exercise. There is strong clinical evidence that Tai Chi has a lot of potential to treating or preventing a wide variety of health problems as well as giving you significant improvement in upper and lower body muscle tone and strength and overall flexibility and balance. There is a growing body of evidence that shows this has an impact on those who suffer from arthritis, ankylosing spondylitis, low bone density and osteoporosis, and even lowers blood pressure and improves circulation, which will reduce the risks of heart disease, hypertension, stroke, multiple sclerosis, Alzheimer's, Parkinson's, stress and a wide variety of other conditions.

Getting started.

Taking a class is the best way to learn Tai Chi. Of course it is possible to learn the movements from a DVD and to a lesser extent pictures in a book, they aren't ideal as you will not be able to appreciate or learn the flow of the movements or the subtle positions of the hands or feet unless you have a teacher there to guide you. Once you are familiar with the basic forms, there is nothing at all stopping you from practicing and exercising anywhere you like. All you need is comfortable, loose clothing and a calm, open space with enough room for you to move, and you are set to go.

If you do decide to take a class, then don't be nervous. Everyone is when they first enter, the strange names, the class full of strangers, the suspiciously tiny powerhouse that could easily throw you across the room teaching the class, it is all a bit nerve racking, but I promise you that soon goes. If you want to observe a class first to see if it is for you, then just ask, any good teacher will be happy for you to do so.

Training.

There are two primary aspects to basic Tai Chi training regardless of what style you train in, entire forms, and individual moves.

Individual moves are just that. Single techniques that are practiced in isolation. In Tai Chi, these individual moves are always practiced with others as part of a flowing form, but essentially the technique must be right first before the form can be considered correct. Tai chi is not just a dance, each and every individual move must be understood in isolation before you can understand its wider purpose in the form. At its most basic, any one individual move will have health benefits similar to any given Western stretching exercise. Slowly leaning onto your back leg might stretch the groin muscle or quadriceps for example. Next comes the internal energy flow associated with each movement. Tai chi is predominantly focused on Chi flow, and each move will either gather and store Chi, or it will move and release it dependent on the need. Finally comes the martial aspect of the movement. This is the final aspect of each individual move that most Tai Chi for health classes ignore, and many practitioners do not even know about. Each movement, as well as enhancing strength and flexibility and promoting energy flow, will be a commencement for a defensive or offensive technique, a small aspect that is often left out of many classes.

Forms are simply a series of movements put together into a specific set, so that the end product is similar to a cross between western dance and a Japanese martial arts Kata. These forms are either short or long, unarmed or armed.

Short forms are the easiest to learn precisely because they consist of fewer individual moves and take less time to perform. These are perfect for beginners who are just getting used to the individual techniques, or even for advanced practitioners who do not have much time and just want a quick workout.

Long forms are quite self explanatory really, they are longer versions of the short forms with many more techniques. The difference can actually be quite large however. Where many short forms last between 5 and 15 minutes, a long form can last for over an hour. Learning the techniques themselves can take years of dedicated practice, so to learn the sequence of techniques that make up a long form can take even longer.

The difference between doing either a short form or a long form are much more intricate than simply time and practice however. Part of the training in Tai Chi involves energy, or Chi, cultivation, and shorter forms have much less energy benefits than longer forms and do not have the same exponential gains in Chi cultivation.

Once a beginner has mastered the unarmed forms, weapons can add an extra dimension to your training. This is where many people get nervous or put off, but there is absolutely no need for this at all. In Tai Chi, weapons such as the double edged sword, the broadsword or the spear for example are not just tools, they are not just something you are holding in your hand to use, they are extensions of your own limb and the purpose of the training is to focus the Chi energy through your body and project it through to the end of the weapon, making the technique much more powerful and the energy benefits much more pronounced.

Aerobic exercise.

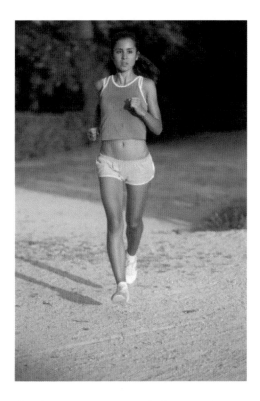

Aerobic exercise is more commonly known by many as cardio. It refers to any type of activity or process that generates aerobic energy, where when you are exercise, your heart beats and you start sweating, and blood pumps more to deliver oxygen to the muscles to keep you moving. Basically, the ability of your heart, lungs and organs to get, transport and use oxygen. Any exercise that you can sustain for a long period of time such as running, jogging, cross training, skiing, anything that gets your heart, lungs and muscles working is considered cardio.

Cardio exercise is essential to living a healthy, balanced lifestyle. It is quite simply a vital component of fitness and health. This is the one stop miracle cure that most doctors and nurses will prescribe to our patients on an almost daily basis.

When we refrain from shouting 'you're too fat! Go for a run!' at someone who is obese and wonders why they have type 2 diabetes and a heart condition, this is what we are referring to. The health benefits should be pretty much self explanatory to most of you.

Cardio exercise is equally as essential as a healthy diet in reducing body fat and maintaining a healthy weight. For those of you who have picked up this book with the aim of losing weight as well as those of you who want to be fitter, then listen up, cardio exercise will be your new best friend. There is overwhelming clinical evidence that shows that cardio exercise is vital to maintaining a healthy weight. It will also reduce your chances of heart disease and stroke, and make your heart stronger, bigger and more efficient. It will lower your chance of type 2 diabetes, perhaps even stop you from getting it if you are warned that you are within the danger zone. It will lower your chances of getting certain cancers and not only extend your life, but improve your quality of life for much longer. It even has proven abilities to help lower depression and dementia! If all this could be turned into a pill, I'd be a millionaire!

The major problem in today's society is sedentary lifestyle. Many of us are far less active now than previous generations used to be. There are many people who have jobs that are not physically demanding, we spend our free time in front of the TV or computer screen, and exercise for many people is still something that they watch those athletes on the TV do. This needs to change, because the lack of general fitness and health in the general population, caused primarily by poor lifestyle choices is causing a huge strain on the NHS.

Current guidelines state that you need to do at least 2 and a half hours of moderate intensity aerobic exercise a week. That is just half an hour a day, 5 days a week. It isn't much time to give up when you weigh it up against what you will gain from doing so. Moderate aerobic activity does not include everyday activities such as housework, for it to be considered at least moderate, you need to do cardio exercise to a level that gets you sweating and out of breath for longer than 5 minutes at the very least. That does mean working hard at it.

Clinical evidence suggests that it is the intensity of exercise that is essential in gaining health benefits and reducing the effects of metabolic syndrome such as diabetes, high blood pressure, high body fat levels and so on. So whilst moderate levels of cardio exercise are good if you are unfit, have never exercised before, or are obese or suffer some other medical condition and need to build up a level of fitness, to really get the health and fitness benefits of aerobic or cardio exercise, you need to kick it up a notch and exercise at a vigorous intensity.

So what counts as vigorous aerobic activity?

Basically this involves a range of activities that get you sweating and out of breath to the point where you can't complete a sentence whilst engaged in it. More technically, this involves getting your heart rate up to 75 - 80% of its maximum. Any type of sport such as football or rugby, jogging, running or swimming fast, aerobics or some sort of cardio class at the gym, all of these and more all count. Exactly which one you choose to do depends entirely on you and what you enjoy doing. There is nothing worse than participating in something you won't enjoy, it just means you are more likely to give up, so choose something that you like and fits in with your individual routine, and stick with it.

How is aerobic fitness measured?

One way aerobic fitness is measured is maximal aerobic capacity, or VO2 max. This is the maximum amount of oxygen your body can consume and utilise, and the measurement of the body's ability to transport and use oxygen during exercise. An average sedentary adult, one with low fitness levels and does very little in the way of activity, can have an oxygen consumption level of 35 millilitres of oxygen for every kilogram of body weight per minute, but elite athletes can have up to 90 ml/kg/minute. Almost three times as fitter as the unfit, sedentary adult. That means someone who is fit can utilise up to three times as much oxygen as someone who is unfit, because they have a stronger heart that does not need to work as hard during exercise, and a larger stroke volume of blood, more efficient muscles and better, more healthier lungs.

There is a very easy way to determine your maximum and resting heart rate, and therefore determine your aerobic fitness. Your resting heart rate is simply how many beats a minute your heart beats when you are at rest, doing nothing. To get your maximum heart rate, subtract your age from 220. This is your estimated maximum beats per minute. Half, or 50% of that number is your lower maximum heart rate. 75% of your maximum number is what your beats per minute should be at moderate aerobic exercise, 85% of your maximum is what it should be when you are engaged in vigorous aerobic exercise. Don't worry, this isn't as complicated as it looks, and you will soon get the hang of it.

You may have heard of the 'fat burning' zone, and for those of you who want to lose weight when they exercise, this seems like a natural target. However, it is a little bit of a myth. There are two types of aerobic exercise, low intensity or moderate exercise which can usually be one over a longer, sustained period such as long distance running, and high intensity or vigorous exercise which is often shorter but more intense such as sprinting. Low to moderate exercise is what people usually mistake as the fat burning zone. This level of exercise occurs when your heart is beating at roughly 60 - 65% of your maximum heart rate, or VO2 max, and it is correct that you will burn quite a lot of calories over an extended period exercising in this way, very slightly more than intense exercise of the same time. However, exercising at 70 - 90% of your maximum heart rate, especially 80 - 85% which is considered high intensity, burns off much more calories overall, and over a much longer period after you finish exercising, because high intensity exercise triggers fat loss by elevating your metabolism for a long time after you finish exercising. So whilst moderate exercise has its place in your programme, intense, vigorous exercise is much better overall at not only increasing your fitness levels, but burning calories.

Types of aerobic exercise.

Running.

Running is what many people picture when they think of cardiovascular exercise, some of them with a sense of dread. A lot of people put off running because of poor fitness levels, they are scared because they normally wheeze when they climb a set of stairs or nearly collapse when they run for a bus, so they put off doing anything about it because it is hard work and they don't want to make a show of themselves in front of other people. This is the exact opposite of what they should be doing!

Okay, running may not be everyone's cup of tea, fair enough. For those people there are a variety of other cardiovascular exercises that can be equally as beneficial. However, so many people actually find they enjoy it once they get into it with huge numbers of people taking part in 5K or 10K runs, or even marathons. Hundreds of thousands of people take part in the London marathon every year, and they can't all be wrong!

Running is ideal for many people because of its inherent simplicity, it is completely free and you don't need an gym membership or fancy equipment if you don't want them, you don't need a partner if you can't find one, and you don't need to put a lot of time in to get a lot of benefits out.

There are different ways to run, either on the treadmill at the gym, or pounding the pavement outside. For some, it is a solitary thing, where they can stick their MP3 player on and forget about the stresses of the world for a while, whilst others enjoy running with others for camaraderie and motivation. It doesn't matter which way you do it, it really doesn't, that is completely up to you. As long as you are getting off your backside and getting fit, then that is the main thing. When you start to burn off that body fat and see the body and muscle underneath all that flab, and you realise that running isn't a chore any more but you actually find it easy to sprint for that bus in the rain, then you will realise it is all worth it.

Getting started.

Footwear is a bit of a bug bear when it comes to training. On the one hand, the correct footwear when running is important, you need a pair of trainers with arch and heel support, anything with flat soles or boots won't do at all. On the other, running should not be expensive, and you shouldn't need to fork out hundreds of pounds for the latest gait analysis and orthotic trainers either unless you have a specific medical problem. For most people, a basic pair of trainers that support the arch and absorb shock to the heel is fine, and the basic ones aren't that expensive.

Measuring how hard you are working during your workout is important, for many people the benchmark of being breathless and unable to talk is fine generally speaking. The technical and more precise aim is to monitor your heart rate and making sure that whilst you are exercising, your heart rate is in the aerobic target zone. This ensures that your heart is working aerobically as opposed to anaerobically, and ensures that you exercise safely. For most people, your heart rate should be between 80 - 85% of your maximum to be vigorously exercising.

The key to starting a real running programme is realistic goals. This is true for any cardio fitness regime really and is pretty much common sense. If you are grossly overweight, haven't exercised in decades, if ever, and find walking to the shops a chore, then it is daft to start out with a programme that expects you to run a mile a minute! Build up to it! Start slow and gradually increase your distance and speed as your fitness improves. It won't take long, and you will feel like a different person.

Most people start running on a treadmill at a gym, and that is absolutely fine. Others prefer running outside. Both have inherent advantages and disadvantages, and maybe it is better to do a little bit of both, but the truth is it doesn't really matter. As long as you are running and getting fitter, healthier and losing that body fat, that's what really counts.

Whichever way you run, it is essential that you bear injuries in mind. Running is a high impact sport, which means that every time you run, your feet are hitting the ground hard and your whole body weight is being forced onto that one spot, this can lead to injuries such as shin splints or knee joint problems, especially if you are running on uneven surfaces such as roads or paths without the correct footwear. Stretching properly is essential. The more flexible you are, the less prone you will be to injury. Rotating your running regime with non impact exercises such as swimming, cycling or cross training is perhaps the best thing to do, as it not only gives your body a rest from the high impact exercise and reduces your chance of injury, but it also gives you the added benefits of those other exercises too.

So how much running do I need to do?

Whether you are training just to lose weight, improve your fitness or for the general health benefits, you will need to meet the challenge of becoming fit head on. This is not the time for excuses or slacking. You don't need to train to Olympic standard, and you don't even need to be that fit to start, just start slow and build up! You will soon see the benefits. This running guide is intended to slowly build up your cardio fitness levels based on how fit or unfit you are at the moment, and should be done alongside flexibility and strength training too, as well as a variety of other cardiovascular exercise programmes. Balance in all things, remember? It is only intended as a rough guide to give you an idea of what you can do, there are plenty more specific programmes out there. By speaking to a personal trainer at a gym and by becoming more familiar with your own body and your own fitness levels, you can get a programme that is very much tailored to your individual needs. Remember that when you start exercising, rest days are just as important, so don't train every single day, it's not good for you, and remember to see your GP or nurse before you start any training so they can advise you based on your own medical history.

Beginners.

Week 1 - Warm up thoroughly. Jog for 5 - 10 minutes at a speed that will get your heart pumping and you out of breath, or your heart rate is working within the vigorous aerobic exercise target. Do this 4 or 5 times a week.

Week 2 - Warm up. Jog for 15 minutes at an aerobic level so you are out of breath. Alternatively run for 30 seconds as fast as you can, walk for 60 seconds and repeat 5 times. Do either one of these 4 or 5 times a week.

Week 3 - Warm up. Run for 15 - 20 minutes at an aerobic level. Alternatively run for 40 seconds as fast as you can, jog for 30 seconds and repeat 5 times. Do either one of these 4 or 5 times a week

Week 4 - Warm up. Run for 20 - 25 minutes at an aerobic level. You should be able to talk comfortably whilst running at this point, but still be out of breath. Alternatively run for 40 seconds as fast as you can, jog for 30 seconds and repeat 6 - 8 times. Do either one of these 4 or 5 times a week.

If you feel that it will take you a little bit longer to progress, or you are finding the level you are at difficult, then don't worry. Just extend the plan for whichever week you are on by another week. If you are not used to exercise at all then it may even take you a week or two to build up to the basic 5 - 10 minute jog. It isn't a problem, just keep it up and you will improve. Remember, it is a marathon, not a sprint! If you have worked your way up through the beginners programme from a previously unfit or sedentary lifestyle, then well done! You should be feeling much fitter and much more alive already. You may even be seeing some fat loss, or at least feeling it!

Intermediate.

Week 1 - Warm up for 10 - 15 minutes. Run steadily for 20 - 25 minutes at 75 - 80% max heart rate. Repeat 4 or 5 times a week.

Week 2 - Warm up for 10 - 15 minutes. Run steadily for 25 minutes at 75 - 80% max heart rate. Or run a mile and a half as quickly as you can. Aim for around 12 minutes. Alternatively sprint for 1 minute, rest for 1 minute, repeat 10 times. Do this 4 or 5 times a week.

Week 3 - Warm up for 10 - 15 minutes. Run steadily for 30 minutes so that you are out of breath but can still talk, or run a mile and a half in 12 minutes at 75 - 80% max heart rate. Do this 4 or 5 times a week.

Week 4 - Warm up for 10 - 15 minutes. Run steadily for 30 - 40 minutes so that you are out of breath but can still talk, or run a mile and a half in 12 minutes or under at 75 - 80% max heart rate. Do this 4 or 5 times a week.

Following this intermediate regime will give you a strong, basic level of fitness. The times for week 3 and 4 are based on the Military's basic selection criteria, so if you can reach them then you know that your fitness levels are basically good. Again, these weeks are only targets, whilst many of you will progress roughly on this timescale if you exercise hard and regularly, don't worry if you don't quite hit that target, just aim for it next week instead.

Advanced.

Week 1 - 10 - 15 minutes warm up. Steady run for 30 - 40 minutes at a comfortable pace but you are still out of breath. Run for a mile and a half in 10 and a half minutes.

Week 2 - Warm up for 10 - 15 minutes. Run steadily for 40 minutes so that you are out of breath but can still talk, or run a mile and a half in 10 and a half minutes or under at 75 - 80% max heart rate. Do this 4 or 5 times a week.

Week 3 - Warm up for 10 - 15 minutes. Run steadily for 40 minutes at 75 - 80% max heart rate. Or run a mile and a half in 10 minutes or under at 75 - 80% max heart rate. Do this 4 or 5 times a week.

Week 4 - Warm up for 10 - 15 minutes. Run steadily for 20 minutes and then run a mile and a half in 10 minutes or under at 75 - 80% max heart rate. Do this 4 or 5 times a week.

Swimming.

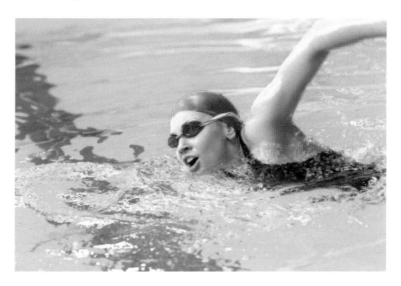

Swimming has a reputation as one of the best all round exercises, and it certainly is deserving of that lofty status. Swimming at the right level, namely so that your heart rate is working at an aerobic level and you are out of breath, not just splashing about in the pool or taking it easy with a breast stroke, holds all the same health benefits as other cardiovascular exercise, plus much more. Apart from running, swimming is perhaps the most efficient calorie burner, it increases your general fitness levels, and exercises and stretches a lot of different muscles all at the same time. On top of that, it is an activity that is available to almost anyone of all ages and sizes, and all you need is to find a local pool and bring along a pair of trunks or a swimsuit and a towel.

Many pools and leisure centres hold classes in the pool with various names such as aqua fit, aqua zumba, aqua fad of the week, that type of thing. For some, they are an absolute bane, as little consideration is given to lanes and half the pool is taken up by what look like wrinkled whales getting in the way and splashing about whilst they are trying to complete their lengths. For others, they are a fun way of getting a little bit of moderate intensity exercise with someone else giving them motivation. To be honest, whilst classes such as these do hold benefits for the elderly, those with joint or mobility problems or those recovering from a joint injury, the aerobic exercise they offer are usually only moderate at best. So if you are swimming for health, fitness and to lose body fat, then getting some vigorous level aerobic exercise from swimming full lengths will be your best bet.

You do not need to spend a great deal of time swimming to get a lot of benefit from it. Just half an hour a day, two or three days a week, combined with a couple of different types of exercise is enough to get your basic exercise requirements. There isn't even any complicated programmes to follow, just swim as many lengths as you can as fast as you can, and keep improving on that target. Swimming is a great way to stay fit for busy people with families too. Take the kids down on a Sunday and turn it into a regular family outing. You'll get fit at the same time as the kids, everyone's a winner!

Cycling.

Cycling is a great, low impact cardio workout that people of all ages and fitness levels can enjoy. Regular cycling is as good as running and swimming at maintaining your fitness levels, reducing body fat levels and the risk of diseases associated with poor lifestyle.

When people think of cycling, they often instantly think of an expensive bike, a skinny guy looking ridiculous in all over lycra and a trendy streamlined helmet, but it doesn't have to be like that at all. Like running, cycling is an activity that can be enjoyed indoors or outdoors, out on the road or in the gym.

Not many of us will need to be taught how to ride a bike, most of us got that when we were kids. Sure, we may be older, larger and flabbier in places now, but get back on that saddle and you will soon be 12 years old again, sticking crushed plastic juice cartons into your spokes to make it sound like a motorbike and relishing in the freedom and the adventure that having a bike brought you before all the boring stuff like growing up and having to be sensible and pay bills took over.

If you choose to cycle outdoors, then you will obviously need a bike. You don't need the most expensive racer or specialist mountain bike unless you really want to advance and train at a high level. For most people, just a basic, relatively cheap bike and a safety helmet will suffice. If you choose to make cycling outdoors a primary part of your fitness regime, then by all means go and get professionally fitted for a bike and shell out a bit more money, otherwise whatever you have will suffice as long as it has two wheels, a seat and a handlebar.

The main thing to remember when you are cycling outdoors is that it isn't just a way from getting you from A to B. It doesn't count if you freewheel downhill all the way to your local McDonalds and reward yourself with a few burgers and a shake! You have to make sure that you are working at 70 - 90% of your maximum heart rate, or 80 - 85% to count as vigorous exercise for at least half an hour. To do this you need to get a constant rhythm going, not coasting every time you hit a downward hill. Try to find a speed that allows you to get roughly 80 pedal strokes per minute.

This can be fairly difficult to sustain sometimes if you cycle on the roads or outside, as you may have to stop for short intervals at traffic lights for example. But even if you don't reach your vigorous exercise target, cycling so that you are moderately out of breath often enough is still great too, and it all adds up.

Cycling indoors on the cycle machines or in spin classes is also a great way of getting fit on the bikes without the problems and hassle of outdoor cycling such as bad weather and irritable drivers. A lot of you may enjoy the social side of spin classes, and if that's what keeps you motivated then that is absolutely fine. Training indoors also allows you to get your pedal strokes much more consistent too, so you can ensure that you are training at the intensity you want to be training at.

Many indoor cycling classes use specific stationary fitness bikes, just in case there were still one or two of you who had never been in a gym and had an image of a load of people carefully negotiating a small room on BMXs. Beyond this the variety within the classes is huge. Some have loud dance music and neon lights, others have fancy projectors with scenes of rolling countryside or coastlines, others still simply have a brightly lit room with a lot of mirrors and an over excited instructor shouting encouragement and instructions at you. To be fair, they are often very good at what they do and can be very motivating.

These classes will often get you working at a good, vigorous intensity, and will have your heart working aerobically at 80 - 85% maximum the majority of the time. The big secret to spin classes and cycling classes is that they use interval training. This is where the instructor will intersperse short bouts of high intensity sprints with harder climbs with more resistance or short periods of slower, moderate exercise, where you will be asked to change position on the bikes at certain periods. This supposedly stimulates the hills and peaks of cycling outside, but more importantly it works. If you are not fit enough to complete a whole class, don't worry, a good instructor will tailor the class to those in it, and allow for various fitness levels. One thing is for sure, you will improve very quickly, and you will soon be pumping away at the pedals with everyone else!

Rowing.

Using a rowing machine at the gym is the closest many of us will get to rowing regularly, which is a shame because it is a fantastic exercise, and quite frankly staring at sweaty people in the gym is never going to be as pleasant as a nice country lake or river! But we take what we can get, and at least we won't get wet in the gym!

The rowing machine offers much more than just great cardio exercise. The aerobic benefits speak for itself, just a relatively short period of intense, vigorous exercise will leave you sweating and out of breath; but it also gives your body a total body workout that will burn a lot of calories because you are utilising more than one major muscle group as well as engaging your fitness levels at the same time. Your whole lower body gets a great workout, because it is your legs that provide most of the power for the drive. But your back, shoulders and arms also get worked hard with the pulling motion of the oar handle, especially if you put resistance on it. Even your core gets a good workout as you fight to maintain correct technique and stability.

Before starting any workout on the rowing machine just as with any exercise, it is essential that you warm up properly. The correct technique is also important when rowing to make sure you don't injure yourself by putting too much strain on the lower back or the knees. If you are a beginner, or even if you have a basic fitness level but have never used these machines before, then start of slowly with no resistance, at a moderate intensity until you get the hang of the correct technique. Remember, if you are ever in doubt, just ask the instructor, that is what they are there for.

Circuit training.

Most people's introduction to circuit training will be in a class at their local gym, but it can just as easily be done on your own with a bit of space and relatively little equipment. It is essentially a pre laid out set of exercises, designed to be done in quick succession in a whole circuit. The amount of times circuits are done depend on the individual, the class, and how many exercises are in any given circuit.

Circuit training is designed to condition the body through strength, or resistance training, and high intensity aerobic exercise that comes with the short intervals between each exercise, and it has been proven to be an extremely effective way of increasing cardio fitness and strength endurance. Circuit training is very easy to set up, and does not even require any equipment in its most basic form, so can easily be done anywhere at any time, in a group or on your own. This ease of use, as well as its adaptability to specific sports has led to circuit training being one of the most enduring forms of aerobic exercise.

The types of exercise vary from class to class and circuit to circuit, but typically incorporate exercises for the upper body, lower body, core and trunk, and total body exercises. Some have specific aims, such as training for strength or training for cardio fitness. Some may even have 'themes' which are popular in modern gyms, and will emphasize different exercises over others, but the fundamentals are the same. Here is a very basic circuit class, designed to be done indoors. You can tailor it, add to it or completely change it as you wish, that is the beauty of circuit training.

Always warm up and stretch thoroughly.

Step 1 - Jog around the hall or on the spot for 1 minute

Step 2 - Do push ups for 30 seconds, followed by burpees for 30 seconds.

Step 3 - Jog around the hall or on the spot for 2 minutes.

Step 4 - Do sit ups for 1 whole minute.

Step 5 - Jog around the hall or on the spot for 2 minutes.

Step 6 - Perform slow squats for 1 minute, with weights if you have them or want to.

Step 7 - Jog around the hall or on the spot for 2 minutes.

Step 8 - Repeat as many times as you need to, twice for a twenty minute workout, 3 times for half an hour and so on.

Fitness classes.

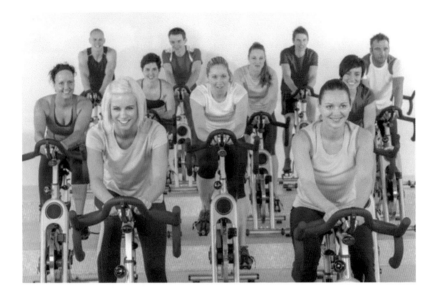

There are a wide range of fitness classes available in many gyms and fitness centres up and down the country. Some of them are fantastic and will give you a great workout in a controlled environment. Many are simply variations on a basic aerobics class based around whatever current trend is popular at the moment so they can lure more fad obsessed people in. Boxercise, aerobacise, Thai Bo, dance fit, zumba, the list is pretty much endless and continues to grow daily as the next popular fad comes in. There is nothing wrong with this in and of itself, but many of them also claim to be things they are not or achieve things they won't. I have heard of one for example claiming that it was the ultimate martial arts workout! But on checking it out, none of the instructors were martial artists, the routines had a vague, passing resemblance to the martial arts they claimed to be emulating, none of the class were doing anything remotely like correct martial arts techniques, and worst of all it was giving the people in the class a false sense of security that they were actually learning how to defend themselves whilst getting fit! As a lifetime practitioner of martial arts myself, this got me a little annoyed to say the least. I'm not saying every instructor is a fake, or that every class is bad, I'm just saying that you have to take these claims with a pinch of salt and check them out for yourself first. Boxercise will not teach you how to box, combat fit will not teach you martial arts, they are in no way a replacement for the real thing, and if that is what you want then it would be better to sign up to a real class and learn the real skill and technique involved in those disciplines.

What these popularised aerobics classes do give you is a great cardio workout. You will get breathless, your heart rate will increase, you will sweat, and you will tone those muscles. Because of the dynamic nature of some of the exercises, you will also often see gains in mobility and balance too. So in that respect these classes are a good form of exercise and I am not disparaging them from that point of view, just don't try and build them up to be anything more than that. The fad sheen they put onto them is just that.

A major benefit of all fitness classes regardless of type is that they are a group activity, and this is something that many people seem to benefit from and enjoy. Don't worry, they really are not the parade of public humiliation and spectacle that some people seem to think they are. No one will drag you to the front of the class and then laugh and point as you start to cry and collapse in a heap because you can't do a star jump properly. Working out and exercising as part of a group can be really motivating for some people, and provide a support structure for both starting and keeping up exercise over the long term. Classes full of people can also take away that temptation to just stop when you start finding the work a little hard going. No one wants to be the first one to collapse in a heap on the floor whilst the rest of the class hasn't even broke a sweat yet, so that will motivate you and push you more, and the feeling you get when you find out you can actually keep up with the class (and that wheezy overweight bloke at the back stopped before you did) is great! There are a great many people who use these classes as a great way to expand their social circle too, and there is absolutely nothing wrong with that. Attending the same class over a period of time may even lead to lasting friendships, and that can only serve to enhance the experience as well as the support factor, mental wellbeing is just as important for a balanced, healthy lifestyle! So if you enjoy these classes, or like the idea of them, and they are the reason that you will get off that couch and get exercising, then go for it!

Fitness classes will also give you the benefit of proper instruction from a qualified fitness instructor in a controlled environment. Like I said earlier, do not expect them to teach you martial arts or how to box, many of these techniques are barely anything more than cardio dance routines that are learned by the instructor, but what you can expect is for the instructor to be fully qualified in fitness, and they will show you how to get that cardio exercise routine right or how to do that sit up correctly, or perhaps more importantly help you on the right path you if you get it wrong, and this is really important for beginners. This specific instruction becomes even more essential when specific equipment is involved, such as the stationary bikes in spin classes, or if you have any injury or pre existing condition, they will be able to tailor the routine slightly for you or may even recommend something different entirely.

One disadvantage to a fitness class is the cost. Now personally I think that your health is absolutely worth it and you should consider the price of a gym membership just one of those bills you have to pay, just like any other direct debit. But I do understand that for many people it will be a concern. If you are not a member of a gym then you will often need to pay either per class or in a bundle, usually a month's worth at a slight discount. Many of them come as part of a membership package though, so provided that you actually use the gym regularly and attend at least a class or two a week, then the monthly memberships can actually work out quite cost effective in comparison.

If you decide that a fitness class is for you, then they really do have a lot of benefits. You just have to pick which type of class is best for you and be aware of what exactly each class involves.

So what type of fitness class should I do?

The exact type of class you choose is totally down to your own particular tastes, interests, fitness goals and availability of each class in your area. Apart from the classes already mentioned such as Yoga, Pilates, circuit training and so on, there are so many different types and varieties, these are just a few of the most popular ones that most gyms tend to have, just to give you a basic idea of what to expect. Remember, your gym may have these exact same classes under a different name.

Aerobics.

Aerobics is a time honoured classic exercise system that has a lot of proven cardiovascular and strength benefits. This is one of those classes that has a wide range of names and styles. Zumba, boxercise, warrior workout, these are all different themes based around the same concept. Some will utilise dancing set to Latin music, others may utilise more upper body punching movements set to a general dance music track or mimic martial arts techniques, all with an instructor at the front of a class yelling out instructions, but all are basically the exact same thing. They are all designed to give you a basic cardiovascular workout that can be set at various levels of intensity depending on your individual fitness levels, and at this they are very effective. Basically expect to raise your heart rate, get out of breath and get a good sweat on!

Aqua aerobics.

You may hear this called aquacise or aqua fit or something similar too. This is essentially the same type of class as a normal aerobics class but set in a swimming pool instead, and is generally a more gentle, weight supported exercise as opposed to the more intense cardio workout of a normal aerobics class. It is a perfect class for a wide variety of people, the elderly, pregnant women, those with injury rehabilitation needs, obese people who would normally struggle with impact training such as running or simply those with a low level of fitness, as the weight supported aspect of the water training provides a mild to moderate cardio and flexibility workout without putting any stress or pressure on the joints.

Abs class.

This is a great class that is obviously designed to concentrate on one specific area that most people are concerned about, your abdominal muscles. These classes have evolved over the years to concentrate more on your whole core area rather than just your abdominal wall, but you will still hear them referred to as abs classes, abs blast, core power, or a variety of other names all designed to make you think you will get a great six pack. The truth is these are great classes for

174

developing and strengthening your whole core area. They are sometimes an hour long, but there are shorter versions which run for half an hour and are billed as intense workouts, and involve the instructor taking you through a variety of sit ups, crunches, oblique twists and others, usually for one minute intervals, to work your whole core.

Body Pump.

This is essentially an aerobic class that concentrates on using light weights and lots of reps to burn fat and build and tone lean muscle. Instructors will take you through a choreographed routine of exercises set to music that utilise free weight plates, a light barbell and a stepper. Instructors are supposed to be specifically trained and accredited to teach this form of circuit class, but in reality it is no different than any other similar class under a variety of different names.

Body combat.

Just like body pump, this is an aerobics class that uses a choreographed routine set to music, but instead of using weights, these routines are simple aerobic workouts that draw on techniques very loosely based on a wide variety of martial arts disciplines. Again instructors are supposed to be specifically trained and accredited to teach body combat, and it bills itself as a martial arts workout, but do not be fooled. Whilst it is an excellent aerobics class that will improve your cardiovascular fitness, the choreographed routines only mimic real martial arts, and are little more than dance routines. There are a huge variety of similar aerobic workouts that are not accredited to the body combat brand, but offer similar aerobic workouts. Warrior workout, combatercise, boxercise, fight fitness and so on, all are variations on the same aerobic theme.

Boot camp.

This is essentially a type of circuit training that is usually, but not always, done outdoors and is based very loosely on a military style full body workout containing a variety of cardio and strength training exercises. Again, the specific style of class will depend on where you go, I have seen variations on this theme ranging from the celebrity boot camp workout (to be honest I have no idea where the celebrity comes into it other than trying to cash in on the fad of vacuous reality shows), to the other extreme of British Military Fitness, where ex soldiers and PTI's will take you through an intensive military style workout in a local park. It goes without saying that the latter especially can be a fantastic cardio workout as well as being great for all over body conditioning.

Crew training.

Imagine a spin class, but with rowing machines. That is essentially what these crew classes are. It is relatively new compared to some of the other classes such as spin, and not every gym has a class in it yet, but it is a fantastic low impact cardio workout that has extra strength benefits for your upper and lower body too.

Spin class.

This is a very popular mainstay of fitness classes, and is found in almost every major gym in some form or another. Most tend to call it spin, or spinning or some similar variation. You use static or stationary bikes in this class, which look like a scaled down version of the indoor cycling machines and allow for a variety of positions and intervals. It is a fantastic high intensity, low impact cardiovascular workout that is great for improving your overall fitness levels and burning body fat.

Your muscles and cardiovascular system get a great workout over changing levels of intensity, which forces them to adapt to the change, without putting strain on your joints. It is set to music, and your instructor will shout out instructions to change the intensity of change your position on the bike at different intervals.

Martial Arts.

There are a wide variety of different martial arts classes available, Karate, Judo, Ju Jitsu, Kung Fu, Tai Chi, Capoeira, fencing and many more. These are not like most of the other classes you will find in the gym, the various martial arts are complete disciplines in and of themselves. Whilst the health and fitness benefits of martial arts are well known and documented, they also offer a lot more than that too. They are complete combat systems with a range of discipline and skill and mental, physical and spiritual development. Taking a class in martial arts can take more commitment than the average fitness class in terms of time and dedication, but can give you much more in the way of improved health and fitness, physical and mental skill and discipline, as well as teaching you a form of self defence and even becoming a way of life for many people.

Zumba.

Zumba is another variation on the basic aerobic workout, this time based on dance, Latin dance specifically, although there have been many variations on this theme. An instructor will stand at the front of the class and take you through the choreographed routine set to music. It really is that simple. It is a class that is suitable for all levels of fitness, as a good instructor will make allowances for different levels in the class, and is a great way to improve cardiovascular fitness as well as burn calories and reduce body fat. There is also an aqua Zumba variation, where a dance routine is performed in a swimming pool. This is essentially an aqua aerobics class with a brand sheen over it. There are many different dance classes out there, not all of them specifically accredited to Zumba, but are equally as good and no different in terms of the health and fitness benefits.

Anaerobic exercise.

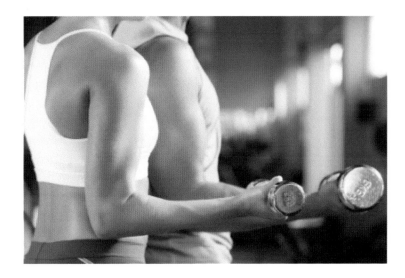

Non endurance sports and exercise such as weight lifting and sprinting use anaerobic metabolism to build strength, speed, power and muscle mass. This is anaerobic exercise, basically strength and muscle training, as opposed to aerobic exercise that utilises muscles which are needed for endurance activities such as long distance running. Any exercise that consists of short, intense movements and powerful exertion is anaerobic.

Just as aerobic exercise is essential in a healthy lifestyle, anaerobic exercise is equally as so. Too many people concentrate on one rather than the other, instead of training in both equally, but this is a mistake. Strength training builds and maintains lean and powerful muscle mass, and on top of giving you that sculpted, shaped body that I know most of you who exercise want, it will significantly will increase your metabolism and make it even easier for you to burn off body fat and maintain healthy levels, it will increase muscle, ligament, tendon and bone strength and density, improving your mobility and risk of falls and injury when you get older. Strength training has many more benefits beside, and combine with cardio training and flexibility can give you that healthy, strong, toned body you have always wanted.

Strength training.

Strength training uses skeletal muscular contraction through weights or other resistance to build the strength and size of your muscles. There are different methods available, weight lifting, either with free weights or machines, or body weight exercises which uses your own body weight as resistance instead of an actual solid weight. Whilst it is essentially training and building muscle, don't confuse strength training with weightlifting or bodybuilding. I know, one seems to go hand in hand with the other, but they are not the same. You can train and build your muscle without becoming huge or bodybuilding.

> Myth Buster! I can't weight train as a woman because I'll bulk up and get muscle! Women especially worry about this, and it simply isn't true. Women do not naturally have the testosterone to bulk up to Terminator proportions. Use light weights and a lot of reps instead to burn more fat, tone up and sculpt your body without building huge muscle. Get the health benefits of strength training and get that bikini body too!

To understand how to build and train your muscle, you must first understand the difference between the two main muscle fibres, namely fast twitch and slow twitch. Slow twitch (type 1) muscle fibres are used predominantly in aerobic exercise such as long distance running. They contract slowly, but have a lot of endurance and can work for a long time without getting tired because they are more efficient at utilising oxygen. Fast twitch (type 2) fibres on the other hand are used during anaerobic exercise or activity for those sudden, powerful movements such as sprinting or lifting something heavy. They are very powerful, but lack endurance. There are also further classifications of fast twitch (type 2a and type 2b) fibres which are a combination of slow twitch and fast twitch fibres and are better at producing sudden, explosive movements respectively.

Whilst body shape plays a large part in an athlete's physique, the best way to picture these different muscle fibres is by imagining the difference between a lean, toned long distance runner or a swimmer, who tend to have a lot of slow twitch muscle fibres, and a bodybuilder, who tend to have a lot of fast twitch muscle fibres. There are different training methods for each muscle type, and the type you train in can determine your body shape to some extent dependent also on your basic body type. An Ectomorph for example will tend to have a muscle composition that contains more slow twitch fibres, and can train these using the right techniques to look lean and toned, but will not be able to get a bodybuilders physique, even by training the limited fast twitch fibres he has. It just means that his core Ectomorph frame will have a limited amount of slightly bigger, more powerful muscles than normal instead of looking lean and trim. Everyone has a different body shape and different muscle composition. It is all about figuring out what your own individual physique is, training for that physique so it is the best it can be as much as it is about what type of training you want to do and the type of body you want to shape. Personally, I think it is best to get a mixture of both types of training to get the benefit of the whole variety of muscle fibres in your body regardless of their natural composition, and make your body as strong, flexible and as healthy as it can be. Body builders almost always neglect their slow twitch muscle fibres, and I see this a lot in the gym with blokes, especially beginners, trying to lift as much as they can as fast as they can. Likewise, there are people who only ever train their slow twitch fibres, but this limits the powerful, fast movements they can do. Like everything else, it is all about balance.

Strength training for different muscle fibres.

Slow twitch muscle fibres.

Cardio exercises such as long distance running will train your slow twitch muscle fibres, and build that toned, lean muscle look that many people crave, but weights and strength training can play an important role too. Using light weights where you can comfortably do a lot of reps or perform a full range of motion with joint movement will tone your muscles and tighten your physique. Aim to be able to do 3 or 4 sets of at least 12 - 15 reps. You don't even have to perform traditional reps, using light weights whilst performing dynamic stretches such as lunges, will make a big difference. Women especially should pay attention here, as one of the biggest myths about weight training amongst women is that they will always put bulk on, and it puts so many of you women off unnecessarily, because it simply is not true! Unless they are using other means to artificially alter their hormone levels, most women do not naturally have enough testosterone to bulk up and train as a bodybuilder. In fact, weight training has been proven to not only burn more fat over a longer period of time, but will get you the body you want once that fat has melted away!

Fast twitch muscle fibres.

Remember, these are responsible for fast, explosive power, so to train these muscle fibres you will need to use heavier weights and fewer reps. Because fast twitch muscle fibres do not have as much endurance, the heavier the weight, the fewer reps you will be able to do. This is the part most men out there will get wrong the first time they set foot in a free weights area. Being able to lift a massive weight and swing it about does not count. You will still need to perform 3 sets of 6 - 8 reps with whatever weight is heavy for you. The specific weight will be different for every individual, but you should be able to lift it and do controlled reps, but be struggling to lift the last rep or two in each set. Over time, this type of strength training will build dense, powerful, bulky muscle.

Mixing it up.

Whilst it is fine to concentrate a large portion of your workout plans to one type or the other, especially if you are doing sports specific training, remember that it is a much better idea for both men and women to train in both types of strength exercise and build up both fast twitch and slow twitch muscle fibres. Combination training like this, alongside mixing it up with cardio and flexibility, is the key to a healthy body.

Understanding reps and sets.

You may have heard the terms reps and sets used quite a lot when talking about strength training or lifting weights, whether it was reading about them in a fitness magazine that told you to do so many of this or so many of that, or down at the gym when you overheard all those blokes bragging about how many they could do. The simple fact is, to do any sort of strength training programme at all, you do need to know what these two terms mean.

A repetition, or rep, is simply one complete exercise such as a dumbbell curl, performed once. How many of these you perform consecutively depends on the weight you are lifting, how strong you are or how long you have trained, and which muscle fibre type you are training. On average, to build powerful dense muscle mass, you need to do 6 - 8 reps with a heavy weight. To maintain and tone muscle, you need to do 10 - 12 reps, whilst 14 - 16 reps with a lighter weight will build toned, lean muscle. Remember, to ensure that you are using the right weight for the type of training, you should be able to lift it properly using good technique and not swing it about, and you need to be able to do all of the reps, but find it difficult on the last couple. Muscular failure occurs when you simply cannot do one more rep, it is like your arm has gone on strike and refuses to do what you are telling it to do, which is lift the weight. Despite the ominous name, this is actually a good thing.

A set on the other hand is a group of repetitions, and on average you should be aiming to do 3 sets of any given number of reps dependent on your training goals, so you could do 3 sets of 10 - 12 dumbbell curls for example. If you are a complete beginner, then it is often better to start with just one set of 10 - 12 reps on each muscle group, and then increase the number of sets to 3 after a week or two once you are used to it.

Types of strength training.

There are different methods available for strength training, body weight training, free weights, and machine weights, and all have their advantages and disadvantages. As always, it is a good idea to get a combination of all of these major types within your wider routine. If you concentrate mostly on free weights for example, then mix it up and have the occasional session where you just use your own body weight or just use the machines. Or better still, have a combination of two or even three in one workout.

Free weights.

Free weights are perhaps one of the best, but for many the most intimidating way to build muscle and develop strength. Unlike isolation exercises that are practiced with machines for example, free weights not only train specific muscles, but often the supporting tendons, muscles and joints too. Often more than one muscle group can be trained at the same time, such as in compound exercises. This means that in general, our entire bodies will grow stronger and more healthy, be much more realistically functional, and more able to cope with the demands of sport or general activity than it would be if we only ever trained our biceps with a machine for example.

Myth buster! Free weights are just for men! Rubbish. Women for some strange reason seem to be afraid of the free weights area, whether they see it as a male only area, or they don't want to use weights because they think they will grow huge muscles. Neither of these things are true. Just come on over, pick up a light weight or a

For some reason a lot of people, especially women, don't want to come anywhere near that small corner in the gym with all the dumbbells and strange bars with heavy weights on them, and it isn't all to do with the strange bloke grunting and making strange blowing sounds when he's lifting something. Although to be fair those people put everyone off. I suspect that most of it is to do with being unsure of exactly what to do with those little bars of metal, but it really does not need to be like that.

The secret to using free weights is technique. Get it wrong, and you could land yourself with an injury, get it right, and you'll build muscle in no time. All you need to do is find yourself the right weight and start doing one of these specific exercises.

Remember, weight in and of itself is not the most important thing. You have to find the right weight for each individual muscle group, instead of trying to be all macho and picking up the heaviest weight you can find because the bloke before you could lift that. Some muscle groups are more powerful than others, your thighs and chest muscles for example, and can lift a lot more than the smaller muscles such as your shoulders, so make sure that you are lifting the right weight for each exercise.

> Myth buster! Free weights are dangerous. No they aren't, with correct training and technique, free weights are very safe. They are only dangerous when used incorrectly or dropped on the floor from a height, which a lot of beginners tend to do.

Bicep curl.

This is one of the most popular free weight exercises because it goes right to the heart of what most men want to build up, their biceps brachii, or their upper arms. It can be done with a dumbbell in each hand or a single barbell.

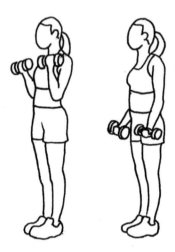

1. Stand with your feet shoulder length apart, your knees slightly bent and your back straight.

2. Holding the dumbbells close to your body with your arms straight, slowly and carefully lift the dumbbells up to your chest so that your closed palms are facing upward.

3. Slowly lower them back to the starting position. You can do this one arm at a time, or both together.

4. For an average workout, do three sets of 10 - 12.

Tricep curl.

This is another popular exercise as it works the back of the upper arm, the tricep, and depending on the weight used, can build strength and muscle mass, or can tone and define the back of the arms.

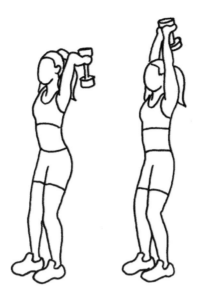

1. Stand with your feet shoulder length apart, your knees slightly bent and your back straight.

2. Raise your arms straight above your head, and slowly and carefully lower the weights behind your head, you should feel the work in your tricep.

3. Slowly lift them back to the starting position. Again you can do this one at a time or both together depending on the weight.

Bent over row.

This is a compound exercise that targets the middle back, the triceps, biceps, trapezius and the rear deltoids, as well as the core to a small extent. You will need a bench for this one.

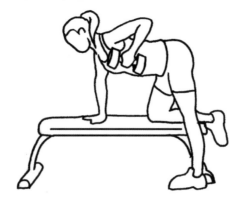

1. Put one knee and one arm on the bench, so that you are half kneeling on it.

2. The weight should be in your free hand, hanging down to the floor, then simply bend your elbow to raise the weight to your stomach.

3. Slowly lower back to the floor and repeat as many times as your reps allow.

Forward shoulder raise.

This works another area popular with men, the anterior deltoids. More specifically, the front shoulder.

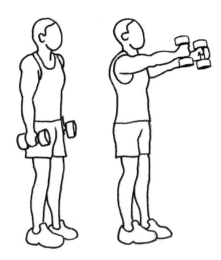

1. Stand with your feet shoulder length apart, your knees slightly bent and your back straight.

2. Hold the weights in front of your hips so the back of your hands are facing forward.

3. One arm at a time, slowly lift your arm in front of you, then slowly bring it back down and repeat with the other arm.

Side shoulder raise or lateral raise.

This strengthens the deltoid muscle and gives you that toned or powerful looking shoulder.

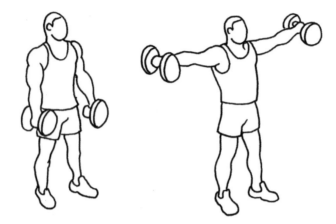

1. Stand with your feet shoulder length apart, your knees slightly bent and your back straight.

2. Do not arch your back or swing your arms up, keep the movements slow and controlled.

3. Hold the dumbbells down at your sides, then slowly raise both arms so you are holding them out to your sides at shoulder level. Slowly lower them to the starting position.

Military raise.

This is a compound exercise that targets the deltoids, the trapezius, the triceps and your core.

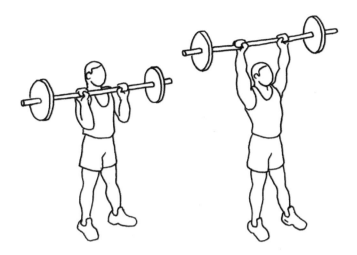

1. Stand to attention with your feet together and your back straight.

2. Hold two dumbbells at shoulder height, with your palms facing forward.

3. Slowly raise both dumbbells above your head, keeping your back straight, then slowly lower them again to your shoulders, keep your palms facing forward.

Bench press.

This requires a flat bench as well as weights. A barbell or dumbbells can be used for this exercise. The bench press works the pectoralis major muscles, more commonly known as the pecs, or chest muscles. This is known as a compound exercise as it also targets the triceps as well as the chest.

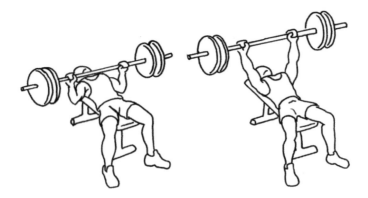

1. Lie flat on the bench with the weights held by your chest. The bar should be across your lower chest if you use a barbell.

2. Slowly exhale and extend your arms upward.

3. Hold the weight for a second, then slowly inhale and bring it back down to your chest and repeat.

The fly.

This again requires a bench, but only dumbbells can be used. The fly works the pectoralis minor muscles, or the smaller muscle in your chest responsible for the rotation, flexion and abduction of the arm.

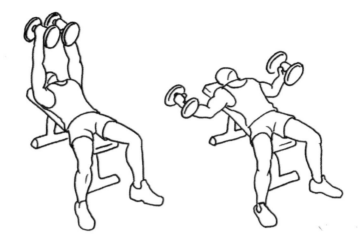

1. Lie flat on the bench and start by holding the weights above you with your arms extended.

2. Slowly inhale and very carefully lower them, keeping your arms almost straight with your elbows slightly bent, until the weights are being held outward at your side.

3. Keep the weights extended away from you and in line with your shoulders, and be very careful not to lower your arms too much.

4. Slowly exhale and bring the weights back up to their starting position. Repeat for 3 sets of 10 - 12.

The weighted squat.

The primary muscle worked here is the quadriceps, or your thighs, but this is another major compound exercise and works all the major muscles of the legs as well as the gluteals, or your backside, your lower back and even your abdominal muscles to some extent. This differs from the squat stretch by adding weights for resistance and working the slow twitch and fast twitch muscle fibres. There are two versions of this exercise, one with the dumbbells held down by your sides, and the other with a barbell held across your shoulders behind your head. Please seek advice from a personal trainer at the gym for this exercise in particular, as you have to be careful to get the technique correct to avoid lower back strain and injury. If you do this with a barbell and you have access to a squat rack, then use it for safety.

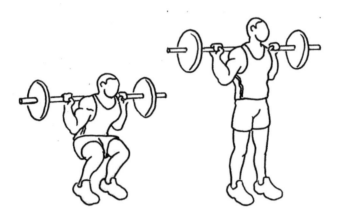

1. Stand with your feet shoulder length apart, your knees slightly bent and your back straight.

2. Lean forward slightly and bend your knees so you lower yourself down.

3. Keep your head up straight so that it feels like you are sticking your bum out and arching your back very slightly.

4. Keep your feet firmly on the floor, and slowly lift yourself back up to a standing position.

Body weight training.

These exercises are a way of getting moderate strength gains similar to weight training, but without using the weights. You use your own body weight and gravity to provide the resistance needed to build muscle, and body weight training alone will not achieve the same results as weight training, although extra weights can be added to provide extra resistance and even greater gains in training the powerful fast twitch muscle fibres.

They are perfect exercises for those on a budget or those who are fixed for time, as on the whole they do not require any money or take up too much time, so are perfect to fit into those spare half hours during the day. They can be done at anytime, anywhere, and are relatively simple.

For some body weight exercises, a basic level of strength and flexibility is required to perform at a basic level. Those unused to exercise or are overweight may find it difficult to perform many pull ups or some of the more advanced abdominal exercises for example, but that basic level can be achieved with a mixture of weight training and aerobic exercise and then the gains you will get from body weight training will increase exponentially.

If you are doing these exercises as part of your normal exercise routine, then that's great, if you are doing them as a workout in and of themselves then don't forget to warm up properly, stretch and cool down just as you would with every exercise. There are a number of different exercises for you to do to exercise every major muscle group.

Push up.

Everyone knows the good old, traditional push up. This is a great compound exercise that works your chest, your arms and your shoulders, and your core to a smaller extent. From a prone position on the floor, you raise your torso up and down using your arms. Simple, right? Try doing ten of them right now! Many people are surprised at how physically demanding push ups get after the first few, unless you are used to exercising and have already got a decent amount of fast twitch muscle fibres in the chest, triceps and shoulders that push ups develop.

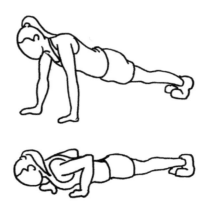

1. Lie on the floor and raise yourself up onto your hands and your toes.

2. Lower yourself so that your body and nose are almost touching the floor.

3. Use your arms to push yourself up.

4. If you are not used to exercise, or are not yet strong enough to do many push ups, the trick is to just try and do as many as

you can for as long as you can. Try to just do 5 at first, then 10, then 15 and so on. Before long, you will be pushing out 3 sets of 30 or more without breaking a sweat.

5. If you do manage to get up to a good standard with push ups, and you want to achieve even greater strength gains and muscle mass, then it is easy to do so by placing your feet on a raised surface or performing it with one arm, Rocky style.

Burpee.

Despite the daft sounding name, this really is one of the classic bodyweight exercises. It has strength gains for almost the entire body, your chest, shoulders, arms, torso and legs will feel like they are on fire after a heavy session, on top of that you will feel like your lungs are collapsing because of the aerobic workout you get from it too. I know it hardly sounds like something any sane person would volunteer to do, but it seriously should be part of everyone's routine.

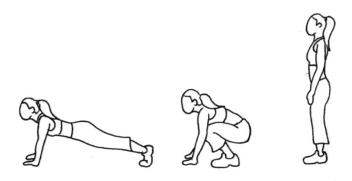

1. Start from a standing position, squat down and put your hands on the floor.

2. Quickly kick your feet back so that you are in a push up position with your arms extended, then immediately jump back to the squat position.

3. Stand up again and jump as high as you can.

4. Just do as many as you can at first, they are really demanding and it might take you time to build up unless you are already fit. Once you are a bit fitter, try and aim to do between 10 and 15 burpees every 30 seconds. This is an ideal exercise to do in a circuit or in interval training, where for example you would do burpees for 30 seconds, then star jumps for 30 seconds and so on.

The dip.

Run on a similar principle to the push up, this compound exercise targets the triceps, as well as the shoulders, chest and back.

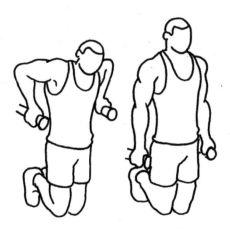

1. Grip two parallel bars which should be slightly wider than hip width apart.

2. Supporting your whole body weight on the bars, keep your arms straight and stiff.

3. Slowly lower your body so that your arms are bent at 90 degrees. This puts a lot of pressure and resistance on the triceps and back muscles. Be careful not to lower yourself too low as this may put too much strain on your muscles.

Pull up.

This is a great exercise to do for the upper body but again is not one that beginners can do without first building up a basic level of strength and endurance. This is another of the relatively few body strength exercises that needs specific equipment, whether that is a specific exercise apparatus at the gym or a chin up bar or something else.

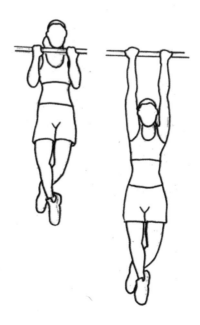

1. Lift your arms and hang off the bar. Your feet should be off the floor and your palms should be facing away from you and have a wide grip.

2. Simply pull yourself up and lower yourself in a slow, controlled manner and repeat as often as you can.

3. An alternative is the chin up. By reversing the hand grip so your palms face toward you and by taking a narrower grip so that your hands are closer together, the same exercise focuses more on the biceps than the back.

Core training.

Core training is a type of training that incorporates many body weight exercises, but one that has developed almost into an exercise system in its own right devoted specifically to your body's core. It has in recent years begun to work its way into popular mainstream exercise vocabulary and has become a bit of a buzz word, go to any gym or fitness centre and you will see at least one class devoted to it.

> Myth buster! Abdominal crunches alone will get me a six pack! Wrong. Even if you had the most muscular torso in the world you won't see it if you are fat. Many people make the mistake of toning up their abs, but then can't see their six pack because of the layer of adipose tissue sitting around their stomach on top of the muscle. You need to lose body fat as well as train the abs to get that six pack!

Many people make the mistake of assuming that the core is just about exercising the abs and getting that perfect six pack. For many people this lean, toned torso and muscular six pack is the holy grail of diet and exercise, and is intrinsically linked to health and sex appeal thank to images in the mass media.

Open up any men's fitness or health magazine or women's gossip magazine and you will usually be inundated with special regimes, diets or plans that will get you that ultimate, sculpted six pack. A lot of them are quite frankly absolutely rubbish, most do not give you the full facts, and this has led to a lot of myths and misinformation about core strength training. First of all any abdominal exercise will not ever burn fat of your belly. It is a myth. A lie. Something told to you by some magazines or fitness websites to get you to part with your money. Quite simply put, spot reduction, where you will see people doing crunch after crunch in order to lose weight and get a six pack, does not work. Secondly, there isn't really any such thing as a six pack either, technically it is an eight pack if anything.

> Myth buster! Lots of abdominal crunches make you lose weight! No they don't. Spot reduction does not work. To lose body fat you have to have a combination of a healthy diet and cardio exercise.

Whilst getting strong abdominal muscles is an important part of core strength, in reality core training is about much more than just getting a six pack. Having a strong core is important for any type of sport or exercise because they allow the transfer of power to the arms and legs and maintain balance, which can even reduce the risk of injury. Imagine your core, your stomach, side and lower back, as your foundation. A weak core means a weak body. Your torso powers all of your movements, it is the source of your stability and balance, keeps you upright, allows you to bend and twist and supports your spine whilst doing so. So the stronger your torso is, the more you will be able to do and the better your quality of life will be. A developed, strong core is equally important in preventing and reducing back pain, and having underdeveloped or weak core muscles, even if you have strong abdominals, is a major contributing factor to lower back pain. Weak core muscles do not allow your lumbar spine to curve properly, will put much more pressure on it and will not support it in giving you good posture.

Core strength refers to your torso, your entire midsection including your sides and lower back, not just your stomach as a lot of people assume. More specifically, the core refers to the muscles that make up the torso, all the abdominal, side oblique and lower back muscles, and those which attach to the spine and pelvis.

The rectus abdominis is the muscle that most people know, the upper abdominal wall. Yes, the one that gives you the 'six pack'. The abdominal wall provides support, protects the internal organs and allows the spine to flex. It is a segmental muscle with eight different parts. This means that if your upper torso moves, the entire abdominal wall is used, but the upper portion is emphasised. If the hips, legs or lower back are utilised, then the focus is on the lower portion of the abs. So to fully train the muscles of the stomach and the front of your torso, you really need to train all of these muscles, and that involves a range of exercises.

The transverse abdominis is the deepest abdominal muscle and lays around your spine for protection and stability. It is like a natural weight belt in a lot of ways. This is the muscle that many people often mistakenly ignore in favour of trying to develop the rectus abdominis which lays above it for that six pack, but this is the real muscle that will give your core true strength and stability.

The external obliques are basically at the side of your abdominal wall. The superficial reason to train these muscles is that they will tighten and tone your torso, specifically the sides, and make your six pack more prominent assuming you have a healthy level of body fat of course. More importantly, they also stabilise your torso and allows it to rotate.

The internal obliques lay underneath the external obliques. They have an important function in the mechanism of breathing, and assist the external obliques in the rotational movement of the torso.

Top Tip! Be careful when doing abdominal crunches during and after pregnancy. After the first trimester you need to be careful about lying flat as this can have an effect on your blood pressure. There are some alternatives however. After childbirth, postpartum abdominal reconditioning as it is known, can cause harm if you are not careful. Abdominal separation is quite common during pregnancy as your bump grows, and loose joints and weak muscle can force limbs or joints out of alignment. Leave any abdominal exercises until 6 weeks postpartum, maybe a little longer if you are personally not ready.

The standard crunch.

Everyone knows the crunch, it is the basic quintessential sit up. There is evidence to show that all abdominal exercises work all of the abdominal wall to some extent, but some exercises work more on the upper or lower part of your abdomen than others. The crunch really targets the upper abdominal wall. There are a lot of different ways of doing this, but the basic crunch is fairly straightforward.

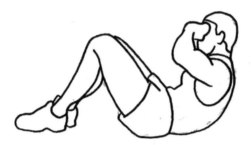

1. Lie flat on your back with your knees bent and plant your feet flat on the floor. Some people find that having someone hold their feet or using a sit up bar is helpful, but it is better if you can do them without.

2. Cross your hands and place them on your chest, or place them lightly behind your neck. Be careful not to pull on your head as you raise yourself up, which can cause strain on the neck.

3. Keep your feet on the floor and your bum and lower back flat while you raise your upper torso up as high as possible.

4. Slowly lower your upper body down to the ground again, but don't let your back fully hit the floor.

5. Lift your upper torso back up again and repeat.

6. If you are a beginner, just try and do as many as you can at first until you can do 10 complete sit ups. When you have

managed that, aim to do 3 sets of 10, and then 3 sets of 20 and so on. Keep it up and you will eventually improve.

The weighted crunch.

This is exactly the same as a normal crunch, but is done with the added weight of a medicine ball or a weight plate held to or by your chest. This is great for adding that extra resistance to your crunches and really developing the fast twitch muscle fibres in your abdominal wall. This can even be done by lying inverted on a steep incline bench which increases the resistance even more.

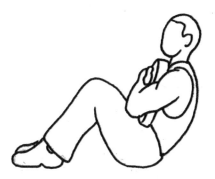

The V crunch.

This is an advanced version of the basic crunch. This is a difficult exercise to do that targets the whole abdominal wall really well, and you may not be able to do this before you can do a fair level of basic crunches, but if you want to make it even harder once you reach an advanced level then you can use a medicine ball to add resistance.

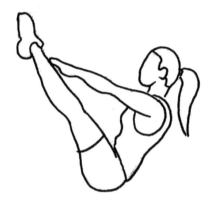

1. Start of in exactly the same way as a basic crunch and lie flat on your back but this time with your legs straight and held together.

2. Lift your torso in the same way as you would a basic crunch, but lift your legs at the same time so that your body makes a V shape.

3. Reach out with your hands and touch your feet when you reach the top of the crunch.

The air bicycle.

This will feel a little bit strange and unnatural at first, but stick with it and you will soon get the hang of it. The most important thing as a beginner is to go slow and concentrate on getting the technique right.

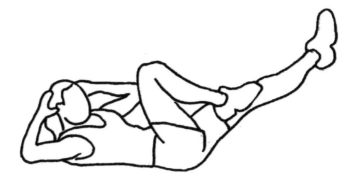

1. Lie flat on your back and put your hands beside your head, again be careful not to grip your head and pull on your neck.

2. Lift your knees up and lift your upper torso up at the same time.

3. Now imagine you are on a bike and slowly move your legs as if they are moving the pedals. At the same time, as your left knee comes close to your body, bring your right elbow up to touch it, and then do the same with the opposite leg.

4. Keep repeating until you cannot do any more. Try and aim for doing 10 at first, then 20, then 30, and keep building upwards.

The leg raise.

This is sometimes called a reverse crunch too. This is a great exercise for focusing on the lower rectus abdominis muscles, basically the lower part of your abs.

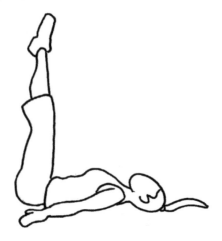

1. Lie flat on your back, either on a bench or on the floor.

2. Put your arms right out to your side for balance or hold the sides of the bench, and hold your legs out straight with your feet together.

3. Slowly raise your legs until they are 90 degrees from the floor, and slowly lower them again without allowing your heels to touch the floor, and then repeat.

4 If you are a beginner, just try and do as many as you can at first until you can do 10 complete sit ups. When you have managed that, aim to do 3 sets of 10, and then 3 sets of 20 and so on. Keep it up and you will eventually improve. Once you reach a proficient level, you can hold a medicine ball between your feet to make it more difficult and add resistance.

Side oblique twist.

This title is almost self explanatory really, it requires a twisting motion to strengthen and develop the side obliques. This really tightens and tones the sides of your torso and is one of the major core exercises that everyone should be doing.

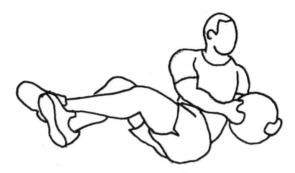

1. For beginners, get in the basic crunch position, on the ground with your feet flat on the ground and your knees slightly bent.

2. Lift your upper body off the ground and hold your hands together in front of you.

3. Tense your abs and slowly twist from side to side, reaching to the floor with your hands on each turn.

4. Once you get used to the basic technique, start using a medicine ball, increasing the weight as you get stronger. Simply hold the ball in front of you, and touch it to the floor on each twist.

5.For an advanced technique, lift your legs off the ground as well as your upper body, forcing the supporting muscles of your torso to keep you balanced as you twist and develop your side obliques.

Oblique crunch.

This again is based on the basic crunch, and is a cross between that and the side oblique twist, so the movement should come quite easily to you if you have mastered that.

1. Lie flat on your back with your knees bent and plant your feet flat on the floor.

2. Put your hands either on your chest or by your head and lift your torso as you would for a normal crunch.

3. Slowly twist your torso to one side before returning to the centre and lowering your torso. Repeat on the other side.

The plank.

This stretches your abdominal and lower back muscles.

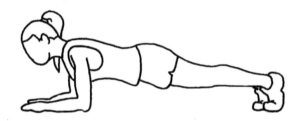

1. Lie down prone on the ground.

2. Use your elbows and toes to lift your body off the ground.

3. Keeping your forearms and palms on the floor, keep your back straight and your head in line with your spine.

4. Gently contract your bum muscles, and hold for 30 seconds.

Back exercises.

Remember that to exercise your core means more than just exercising your stomach, you need to support your lower back too. Developing strong back muscles is absolutely essential to living a healthy lifestyle, as anyone who has ever suffered a back injury will tell you. Even a minor back strain or injury can be crippling and put a serious strain on your lifestyle in more ways than one. This is why training your back, especially your lower back, is so important. There are strength training exercises for your lower back that you can do too, but many of the exercises that involve your lower back are stretches. These are some of the more popular examples. As with any exercise care must be taken with correct technique so as not to put too much strain on your spine or injure your back.

The Superman.

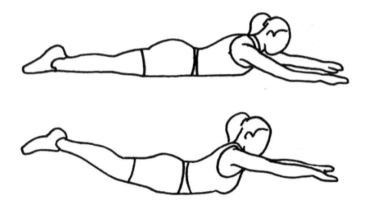

1. Lie face down on the floor, with your arms extended in front of you.

2. Exhale slowly and lift your arms, your legs and your chest off the ground at the same time. Squeeze your lower back.

3. Hold for 3 seconds and then lower yourself to the starting position.

4. Repeat as many times as needed.

Cat stretch.

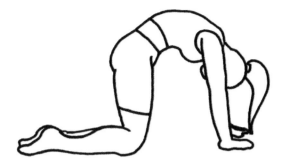

1. Start by leaning down on all fours, your palms should be shoulder length apart and facing the same direction, and the tops of your feet should be on the floor. Your knees shouldn't be too far apart either, try and get them in line with your hips.

2. Keep your head lifted so you are looking down to the floor but your head isn't hanging down.

3. With a slow exhalation, slowly arch your spine upward. The spine should be the only part of you that is moving.

4. Imagine each and every segment of the spine separating and stretching as you move, lower your head slightly at the same time.

5. As you inhale, slowly come back down to the starting position.

Hyperextensions.

Hyperextensions are a great exercise for targeting your lower back. They can be done in one of three ways, either with a specific hyperextension bench, a normal bench with a partner holding your legs, or a specific back extension machine with weights. The movement and exercise is essentially the same, it's just a case of personal preference and what equipment you have available.

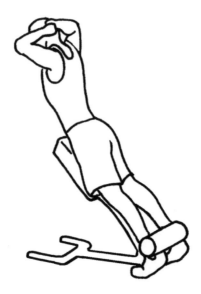

1. Lie on the bench and secure your ankles, make sure the bench is adjusted properly so that the edge lies against the front of your hips and you can bend forward without restriction.

2. Cross your arms on your chest and lower your torso to roughly 90 degrees from your legs. Be careful not to bend too much and bend your back.

3. Raise your torso until your back is straight, be careful not to overextend your back as this may cause too much strain.

4. Repeat as many times as your reps and sets allow.

Exercise and pregnancy.

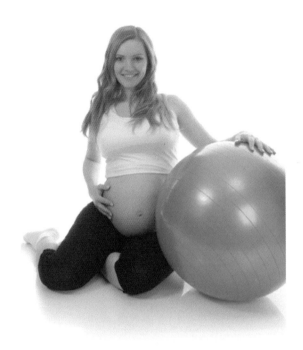

Is it safe to exercise when I am pregnant? This is an extremely common question asked by many women before and during their pregnancies, and one with a very simple general answer, Yes, and a more complicated longer answer that generally fluctuates around the catch all term 'within reason'. Don't worry, I'll walk you through exactly what you need to know, whether you have never done any exercise before in your life, or you are an Olympian athlete who suddenly finds yourself in uncharted territory.

It is essential of course that before starting any exercise or continuing with your regular routine, you must first speak with your midwife or your physician, who can give you much more specific advice than this book can based on your own particular medical history and individual needs. There are a number of medical conditions such as pregnancy induced high blood pressure, cardiac, vascular or pulmonary disease, an incompetent cervix and a previous history of problems during pregnancy for just a few examples, that you will need to discuss with your midwife or physician before you start. In general though with a few slight modifications to types of exercise or routine, exercising is not only safe, it is actually beneficial to both you and your developing baby.

The general consensus based on a lot of clinical study is that mild to moderate exercise is best throughout pregnancy, so if you were planning on running a marathon, don't! Stick to relaxing flexibility exercises, mild to moderate cardio workouts and some mild to moderate body weight exercises. The emphasis here is on mild to moderate exercise that makes you feel good and maintains your fitness, not exercise to prepare for a gruelling event. This is why it is also essential to remember your rest days! Take it easy. I know you all hate being treated like an invalid, especially in the later stages of pregnancy when you should have everyone running round you fearful of the ever present threat of you turning into the girl from The Exorcist, but you do need your rest too! It is important! Make the most of it, because you won't get any when the baby is born!

Your body will obviously change quite a lot during your pregnancy, you will have the weight gain, which is absolutely normal but will put extra strain on your joints and lower back and probably aches and pains in parts of you that you never even knew existed. You will have the morning sickness, the hormone fluctuations and many more wild and weird changes which may have many of you wondering what the hell you have gotten yourself into, and this can take a lot of adapting to. The truth is more exercise you do, and the fitter you are before and during your pregnancy will help with this, and certain exercises may help make childbirth a little easier too.

First Trimester.

What exercises should I not do?

It is important to remember that exercise has now been clinically proven to be beneficial to both you and your baby throughout pregnancy and childbirth, but there are a few certain provisions and changes that should be made. Obviously as your pregnancy progresses, you aren't going to be able to do all the same types of exercises and workouts that you did before.

The frequency and moderation of your effort levels are only one thing to consider. If you are completely new to any form of exercise at all then take it easy. Start slow and keep it relaxed. If you are a regular at the gym or you are one of those people who get frustrated if you are not running a marathon or climbing Everest, then tone it down! That's an order! Keep any exercise mild to moderate, it is all about balance.

It is important too that as your pregnancy progresses, especially after 16 weeks, that you do not lie flat on your back to do any exercise. So this means making modifications to any abdominal workouts, yoga or Pilates classes and anything else that may require you to lie on your back. It is okay at first, but just bear in mind that laying on your back to exercise is something you should start phasing out.

Obviously contact sports are out, so no boxing or martial arts or anything that may risk your bump being hit or compressed. Abdominal trauma of any kind is absolutely the last thing you need. Don't worry, the occasional random act of violence against the man that did this to you can be overlooked. It is also important to minimise risk wherever possible too, so no extreme sports or off road cycling! Especially after 16 weeks! Your body will change, and with it your weight, shape and centre of balance too, so this is not the time to take up sky diving, horse riding or off piste skiing! Anything that involves balance, or high impact exercise is out.

It isn't just the type of exercise but the reasons for it that you have to be aware of too. Maintaining health and fitness, improve muscle strength and flexibility, especially in the all important areas involved during childbirth, relaxation and stress release, these are all great reasons for exercising during pregnancy. Losing weight is not. This is an absolute no go area. I know losing weight is a prime reason many of you started exercise or want to start it before you were pregnant, and that is fine, but this should not be your focus now. You will gain weight when you are pregnant, this is absolutely normal, so just accept it. Concentrate instead on the reasons above, as well as maintaining a healthy body image, and the weight gain won't seem as bad. You can always focus on that after the baby is born, and by exercising the right way now, you will find losing weight a lot easier then!

These may seem like common sense now when you think about it, but it is still important to be aware of what you can do, what you have to modify, and what you absolutely can't do at different stages of your pregnancy, especially if any of these things were a normal part of your life before you were pregnant. This self awareness will be one of your biggest allies

222

as you progress through your pregnancy. Even if you are exercising as you should be whilst your pregnant, it is obvious that if you experience any form of discharge, especially bloody, dizziness, pain, elevated heart rate or blood pressure that does not go away, or anything else that you are worried about, then stop immediately and talk to your midwife or GP. It is always better to err on the side of caution.

So what am I allowed to do?

More than you think really. During the first trimester not much has to change at all. Despite some obvious limitations placed on you, exercise is still an essential part of living a healthy lifestyle and having a healthy pregnancy alongside a balanced, healthy diet and plenty of rest. The secret is modifying a lot of what you would normally do to incorporate your pregnancy.

The exercises that you should be doing can be put into two basic categories, the ones that you should be doing any way to maintain general health and fitness such as cardio, and ones that you may need to modify or even start doing such as yoga, Pilates, flexibility exercises and pelvic and core strengthening exercises, that can help your pregnancy become much easier by making you much stronger and flexible in the areas that need it.

Cardiovascular workouts are an essential part of everyday health and fitness, and there is absolutely no reason why they shouldn't be while you are pregnant too. If you are used to exercise, then stick to your normal routine, just slowly start to tone it down to mild to moderate intensity over the next few weeks. If you normally run a few miles and then hit the weights machines for example, then start jogging for a couple of miles and easing up on the weight or resistance you are using. I'm not telling you to stop, just start to tone the intensity down. Many women use the perceived level of intensity for this, which is a simple scale where 0 is no effort at all, and 10 is flat out. You should be aiming for around 6, maybe push it to a 7 during the first trimester.

Basically if you are a beginner, then keep all aerobic workouts to a low intensity level. For those who are already used to exercising then a moderate level of intensity is fine, but still make sure you don't over exert yourself. You should be very slightly out of breath but still be able to hold a conversation with the person next to you. You have to be careful that you don't raise your core temperature too much as this can negatively affect your baby, who is already slightly warmer than you are, and if you get too out of breath too often, then you are using up all the available oxygen instead of allowing it to get to your baby.

Strength workouts will need to start getting easier too. You can still do everything as normal, including lifting weights, resistance training, sit ups and crunches, during the early part of your first trimester, but as with your aerobic workouts, you will need to start toning a lot of these down as your pregnancy progresses. Whilst they are okay to do at the start of and during this first part of your pregnancy, by the end of your first trimester you shouldn't be doing abdominal crunches, planks, or anything that involves you holding your breath or exerting a lot of force.

There is no reason that you can't carry on exercising your muscles throughout your pregnancy, some of them are really important too. Just remember the golden rule, if you are straining to lift it, it's too heavy. Stick to light weights and lots of reps. Just keep thinking of that baby you'll be holding when you are doing the bicep curls!

Exercising your pelvic floor will be essential. Your pelvic floor as most of you will know is one of the most important muscles to consider during your pregnancy, yet one which many of you may have neglected up until now. Don't worry you're not alone, after all, talking about building that perfect beach six pack has a much nicer ring to it than building a strong beach ready uterus and bladder! No matter, it is never too late to start.

The pelvic floor is almost like a cradle that holds your uterus, bladder, bowels and other pelvic organs. Normally in most people there is no problem with this, but during pregnancy your uterus will grow, and your pelvic floor will stretch and weaken. This leads to a host of obvious problems. The main muscle to be concerned about is the Pubococcygeous muscle, that small bow tie (ish) shaped muscle stretched between the urethra, your vagina and your rectum. Not very pleasant, I know, but it is important so stop pulling that face.

The good news is there are a lot of exercises that can help you strengthen this muscle, and these will not only help to stop any of the problems associated with a weak pelvic floor, but can really help ease childbirth too because it will be much stronger and more supple when your baby starts coming out.

Core exercises are absolutely essential during pregnancy too, as a strong core will support the added weight of the baby and help prevent back pain, and can also support the uterus during actual childbirth, making it easier. Don't worry, I know a lot of women worry about this but you will not harm the baby. You do however still have to be really careful. Your core, if you remember from the previous section, is your whole torso, your stomach, your sides and your back, and consists of the internal and external obliques, the rectus abdominis and the transverse abdominis amongst others. These muscles, as well as your lower back muscles, form a girdle of sorts around your core, they keep everything tight and secure, and will really assist your pregnancy and your birth if they are strong enough. During the first trimester, a normal routine should be absolutely fine. The core exercises described in the previous section are absolutely okay to do, provided that you keep the intensity to a low to moderate standard.

Flexibility workouts are perhaps one of the best all round types of workout that you can do throughout all stages of your pregnancy. Your body will go through a lot of changes that will put a lot of pressure on your spine, joints, tendons, ligaments and affect your posture. The more flexible you are the more effectively you will be able to adapt to and cope with these changes both during your pregnancy and during your postpartum period.

The majority of the flexibility exercises in the last chapter will be more than sufficient to ensure that your body stays in the best shape it can during your pregnancy, and will give you added benefits in stress reduction and time that can be set aside for meditation or just for you without any interruptions. With minor modifications, such as not performing any of the poses that require you to lay flat on your back, then yoga and Pilates, Tai Chi too are absolutely perfect during and after pregnancy. Just keep in mind that especially after the second trimester onward, mild to moderate effort should be given only, do not try and push any moves or stretches that you find uncomfortable, or perform any techniques that will put too much strain on you, especially if you are not used to it. This is why it might be a good idea to train with a qualified instructor in a class, especially if you usually train alone. If you go to a class, particularly if you have never been to one before, make sure that you let your instructor know that you are pregnant. That way they can alter your workout and advise you as necessary.

Second Trimester.

What exercises should I not do?

At the start of your second trimester, this is when things really start to change. Your bump will start showing soon, but all the annoying morning sickness will be easing up at least. This is when you need to start making definite changes to your workouts

At the start of your second trimester, it is strongly recommended that you do not lie on your back to exercise at all, as this puts a lot of pressure on the vein known as the superior vena cava and can reduce blood flow to your heart, and perhaps even your brain and uterus. Obviously this will not be the case for all women, but as always, why take the risk? You also don't want to do any plank or excessive crunch movements either so the core exercises that you do, whilst being predominantly the same or similar to what you would normally do, should be modified slightly to incorporate those factors.

Diastasis recti abdominis.

As you progress in your pregnancy, your bump will obviously grow. This means your abdominal muscles will weaken and soften thanks to your hormones, and then stretch and sometimes separate, which can lead to a relatively common condition known as diastasis recti abdominis, or abdominal separation, where the right and left sides of your rectus abdominis, or your six pack muscles get pulled apart at the linea alba, the thin connective part that runs right down the middle of your abdomen, (that little line you see in the middle of the six pack abs). Don't worry, as I said it is quite common and is only temporary, it usually goes away after you have given birth and the abdominal muscles return to normal. A strong core before and during pregnancy will help prevent this, as will performing the correct exercise and obviously avoiding the incorrect exercises, during pregnancy.

To test if you have abdominal separation, then simply lie on your back and put three fingers together, place your middle finger an inch above your belly button and then do a small, gentle crunch as you press your fingers gently into your stomach. If all three fingers feel as if they are sinking into a gap, then your muscles have separated.

If you do have, or get diastasis recti, then don't worry. Remember it is common, you will just need to modify the core exercises that you do so that the condition doesn't get worse and so you don't cause yourself harm. Normal abdominal exercises like the plank, any twisting side oblique exercise, traditional crunches, these are all out. Stick instead to flexibility training and stretches.

So what am I allowed to do?

Walking is an ideal form of cardio exercise, either on the treadmill or outside, particularly for those of you out there who have never done a day's exercise in your lives (you know who you are!) For those of you who are a little fitter, then walking at a pace that will get your heart rate comfortably up and you are breathing more quickly, but not so much that you can't talk normally is still easy to do, and can be done anytime throughout the day. Even simply walking to the shops counts as exercise.

If you are already fairly fit, then jogging to maintain a level of fitness is absolutely fine too to an extent. Just listen to your own body and don't push yourself too hard. If the pressure on your lower back or your joints becomes too much once you start gaining weight, then stop, and remember do not be tempted to knock the speed up on the treadmill or push yourself that little bit further. You should be aiming for a perceived intensity level of about 5 out of 10, which means you should be able to talk comfortably as you exercise.

Swimming is also a fantastic exercise. That reputation for being one of the best all round exercises didn't come from nowhere. It can give you that mild to moderate workout easily and enjoyably so you are not exerting yourself too much. It is also important to consider that as your pregnancy progresses and your body changes during the second trimester, you will have added strains on your back, spine and joints already. Impact exercises like running or high energy dance and fitness classes may become impractical, so swimming allows you to carry on exercising whilst supporting your body and removing all that extra pressure and strain.

Strength exercises are still fine to do during your second trimester, but if you normally lift a moderate to heavy amount of weight, it will be a good idea to start easing up on that now. All those extra strains and pressure on your spine and joints from your rapidly growing bump doesn't need to be compounded by heavy weights! Light to medium weights are absolutely fine though, just remember to listen to your body and do not strain yourself. Seek advice from the trainers in the gym if you want a variety of exercises for lighter weights.

Using equipment such as kettlebells are great too, as they will provide you with the strength and mobility exercise you need and allow you to focus on specific areas such as your lower body, legs and abdominal muscles. This will improve your balance, posture and stability without putting too much strain on you. Just remember that as with any type of exercise during this period, concessions must be made, so avoid any of the exercises that involve jumping, quick movements, high impact or put too much strain on your lower back. As with everything, keep it moderate too. You should get a good workout by all means, but from the second trimester onwards, do not push yourself to the point of exhaustion. Consult with the trainers at the gym to get a range of specific Kettlebell or medicine ball exercises that will be safe and easy to do during this period.

It is very important that you keep up your core and pelvic floor exercises, the benefits during and after childbirth will be more than worth any effort you put in now, believe me. The only difference is in the type of core exercises you should do. Your body will be different, so it makes sense to adapt your training, right? Remember that you should not be lying on your back for any of these exercises now, and you shouldn't be doing crunches either. But there is a variety of exercises you can do.

The first thing you should do is get to know the stability ball, that huge rubber thing usually sitting in the corner of the mat work area in the gym gathering dust, you may even have one sitting in your spare room with ironing strewn all over it. Get it out, it can be your best friend while doing these exercises, especially when your bump starts growing and doing normal abdominal exercises become uncomfortable. These balls are known by a dozen names or more, fitness balls, stability balls, Pilates balls, Swiss balls, balance balls, they are all essentially the same thing. I have no idea why they have so many different names, other than people wanting to market their own brand of exercise I suppose, but either way it doesn't matter. These can be used for a whole variety of exercises and are essential for doing core exercises when you are pregnant, because they take you off the floor and remove the associated negative health effects, and they position you much better for exercising as your bump grows, as well as providing more comfort. It is important though to get the right size of ball for you as an individual, there is no point in getting the small sized ball if you are over six foot, and vice versa.

Standing front to back pelvic tilt.

This is a great exercise to do during your third trimester, and many women find it quite comfortable. Simply stand in a neutral position or with your back up against a wall, whichever is the most comfortable for you. Your feet should be shoulder length apart and your knees very slightly bent and relaxed. If you are standing against the wall, ensure that the back of your head, your shoulders and backside are touching the wall, but the arch of your lower back is not. Now perform the pelvic tilt. Exhale slowly and move your tailbone downwards as you bring the pelvic floor forward, this should cause the arch of your back to curve and touch the wall. Then slowly inhale and reverse it, bringing the tailbone up and arching your lower back. This should be the only part of your body that is moving, and make sure you do not over extend or exert the movement, only do it as far as it is comfortable.

Stability ball front to back pelvic tilt.

This is essentially the exact same exercise as the standing pelvic tilt, except you will be sitting on a stability ball to perform it. Sit on the ball so that you knees are bent at 90 degrees and you are very slightly off centre on the ball. Your tailbone should be supported. Your feet should be shoulder width apart and your spine should be in a relaxed neutral position. Exactly the same as in the standing movement, Exhale slowly and move your tailbone downwards as you bring the pelvic floor forward, this should cause the arch of your back to curve and the ball to slowly roll toward your feet slightly. Then slowly inhale and reverse it, bringing the tailbone up and arching your lower back.

Stability ball pelvic rotation.

This is a very easy exercise that you can do to work the pelvic floor even in the last trimester of pregnancy if you find it comfortable, and many people do. Simply sit on the stability ball and roll very slightly forward, so that your legs are bent and you can feel your quadriceps taking the pressure. Your back should be straight and your spine should be in neutral position. Keep your upper body still and place your fingertips on your hips, now rotate your hips in a very small circle making sure that the rotation initiates from the pelvic floor.

Stability ball incline pelvic tilt.

Lie on the ball so that your middle and upper back and shoulders are on the ball and your legs are bent. Your lower back and hips should be off the ball. Relax your shoulders and your neck. Exhale and use your abdominal muscles to lift up your hips, but don't overarch your spine. Inhale and lower your hips to the starting position.

The stability ball crunch.

This is done exactly the same way as a basic crunch, but is done on the stability ball. Make sure you are positioned correctly on the ball, where the ball is pressed on your lower back. Bend your knees, then slowly lie backward. The ball should still be firm against your lower back and you legs should be bent at roughly 90 degrees. Lift your upper body so that your abdominal wall contracts, then slowly lie back and repeat. This not only builds the main abdominal wall, but also the side obliques to a small extent as well as other stabiliser muscles as you keep your balance. This can also be done at the same time as a pelvic tilt, so you are working the two muscles at the same time. In the first trimester, it is fine to do about 15 reps of these, or less if you find them uncomfortable, and gradually do less as your pregnancy progresses.

The stability ball oblique crunch.

This is another pretty straightforward one. Lie on the ball so that one side of your torso is on the ball and you are supporting yourself with your forearm. Stagger your feet so that your bottom leg is in line or very slightly forward from your body, and your top leg is behind you. This will help you with your balance. Some people also find it easier to put your feet against a wall for even more stability. Place your other hand behind your head and slowly exhale as you lift your upper body up so that you can feel your side oblique contract. Lift with your core muscles, and don't push up with the elbow that's on the ball, that defeats the object. Exhale as you lower yourself down and straighten your torso. Then turn round and repeat on the opposite side. In the first trimester, it is fine to do about 15 reps of these, or less if you find them uncomfortable, and gradually do less as your pregnancy progresses.

The stability ball seated single leg raise.

Sit down on a stability ball and put your feet flat on the floor and hip width apart. Keep your spine neutral and your upper body still. Place your hands on your hips for balance. Slowly inhale and lift one leg off the floor as high as you can, hold for 5 seconds and keep your torso straight and balanced, then exhale and lower your leg to the floor. Repeat with the opposite leg and try to do 15 repetitions on each leg.

The seated double leg raise.

Sit on the edge of a chair so that your backside is fully seated but your legs are not touching the chairs surface and hold the sides with both hands. Lean back very slightly without curving your spine and lift your feet off the ground. Slowly inhale and raise your legs as high as is comfortable, then slowly exhale and lower them without letting them touch the ground. Try and repeat for 15 reps.

Side plank.

This is one that doesn't require a stability ball, but should be comfortable to do at all stages of your pregnancy. Lie on one side and raise yourself so that you are leaning on your forearm. Your elbow should be directly below your shoulder. Just rest your other arm along the side of your body. You can bend your knees so that your feet are behind you if you wish, but your knees, hips and shoulders should all be straight and aligned with each other. Hold this position for 30 seconds and repeat for 10 reps.

Back muscles

The back is as important a part of your core as your six pack is, and during pregnancy your lower back will come under a lot of strain. You are after all carrying a huge extra weight around your stomach. This is why ensuring your back muscles are as strong as they can be will really pay off once your bump starts showing.

Flexibility training, yoga and Pilates workouts that have been modified to take out the mat work aspect of the classes so you do not lie down can be perfect for exercising your back. Obviously traditional techniques which involve lying on your stomach are out too, but there are a variety of back stretches that can be done whilst kneeling down or standing up. The cat pose or the baby pose for example.

Squats.

Squats are excellent for strengthening your lower back, your thighs and your buttocks, all areas which will come under a lot of strain during pregnancy. Squats, alongside core exercises and flexibility training should help relieve a lot of the pain and pressure in your lower back during the later stages of pregnancy. Exercising your quadriceps and major leg muscles may even help you during childbirth if you choose to deliver in a squatting position. If you find it easier, you can do these exercises with a stability ball against a wall, but whichever technique you choose, be careful of knee injury. If you feel any discomfort at all, just stop.

Third Trimester.

What exercises should I not do?

This is obviously the stage where you will be at your heaviest and your bump will be as large as it is going to get. You may be getting a bit fed up of it at this point, but if you have followed the advice in this book, eaten a healthy, balanced diet and continued to exercise in the right way, then you should be feeling a lot better about yourself and you will be a lot more prepared for the demands of childbirth, physically at least anyway. In this stage it is still absolutely safe, even a good idea to carry on exercising, providing that you are still consulting your midwife or physician and there are no medical conditions that would negate it, but you still need to take precautions.

Exercises that involve a lot of jumping about or bouncing, aerobic or dance classes for example, can be uncomfortable and impractical during the third trimester. Running, jogging and cycling can carry increased risks too, especially outdoors on an uneven surface. So if your exercise routine has up until now included high impact exercise, even if you scaled it back during your second trimester, now is the time to limit it even more. Obviously everyone is different and for some women some mild impact exercise may be fine in small doses, but for many it will be a good idea to stop this type of exercise completely.

So what am I allowed to do?

It may sound like I am advising you to stop everything I told you to do in your previous Trimesters and treating you as an invalid, but that really isn't the case. I've been around pregnant women and I'm not suicidal enough to do that! As with the second trimester, it is just a matter of scaling back and modifying your routine to incorporate your changing body shape.

Low or no impact cardio exercises are still absolutely fine to do. Swimming again is the perfect example. Swim to your heart's content. You can swim throughout your third trimester without having to worry at all about your increased weight, changing centre of gravity or any extra pressure on your ligaments and joints. I told you that reputation for one of the best forms of exercise was well deserved!

Using a treadmill to walk on where you are still getting slightly out of breath is generally okay too, if you find it comfortable. Cross trainers or stationary bikes again can be okay, if you find them okay to use. This is the part where it gets a little difficult to advise you in a book, and you have to use your own judgement a little bit. The no impact aspect of these machines are great, and because they are fixed machines, you don't have to worry about your shifting centre of gravity or changing shape because you won't lose your balance on them the same way you would on a mountain bike outdoors for example. So provided that you scale back the intensity that you where using in your second trimester so you don't get too out of breath or overexerted, then they can be absolutely fine to use. However, depending on your actual size and shape (I'm making no judgements, put the sharp objects down), some women may find these machines uncomfortable to use. If you do, just stop. Stick to swimming and walking.

If you have been lifting weights during your pregnancy (and if you haven't then why not?) then there is absolutely no reason to stop now. Lifting weights is absolutely safe during your third trimester, just stick to the golden rule of using light weights that tone your muscles, and do not over exert yourself. If you find it difficult to lift a weight, then it is too heavy, and you will be putting extra stress on tendons and ligaments that have already been weakened by your pregnancy.

It is also important to keep up with your flexibility exercises and your core and pelvic floor exercises too. Again it is safe to do all of these exercises throughout your third trimester, you just need to change or modify what you do. You obviously haven't been able to lie on your back since the start of your second trimester, and now some of you may be finding it uncomfortable to do some side to side pelvic tilts too, but that still doesn't mean you can't do a forward to back pelvic tilt, either standing or sitting on a stability ball. You can perform exercises kneeling down on all fours, but many women find this uncomfortable as the extra weight of the baby adds pressure to the spine. Just be careful and judge what is best for you. If it feels uncomfortable, then stop.

Exercising after childbirth.

Once you have given birth, you may look down at your body and want to get back to a slim, toned midriff as quickly as possible. Don't worry about it so much, just concentrate on letting yourself rest and heal for the first month or so. Leave any actual abdominal exercises until 6 weeks postpartum, maybe a little longer if you are personally not ready. Everyone is completely different and individual, so there is no set time frame, only you can say when you are ready. When you do feel up to exercising again, you can get back to your normal training regime, or follow the advice given in the previous exercise section. Just remember to take it slowly at first, have a few exercise sessions to begin with that are nice and easy at a mild to moderate intensity just to ease yourself back into things. Once you are ready to start exercising normally again, there are some specific exercises you can do.

On top of all the other core exercises and crunches you will undoubtedly do, concentrate on your transverse abdominis too. Exercising your transverse abdominis is often overlooked when women are trying to tone up after giving birth, to be honest it's often ignored by everyone during most abdominal exercise routines, but it really shouldn't be. Imagine your transverse abdominals as the girdle around your torso, these exercises are the strap to pull that will pull that girdle in and squeeze and tighten your entire middle section.

The girdle squeeze.

Start by lying on the floor with your knees bent and your feet on the floor. Press the fingertips of both hands into your lower abdomen. Keep breathing slowly and steadily throughout the exercise. Draw your lower abdomen toward the floor, as if you are tensing the lower abdomen only, but keep the rest of your body still. You should feel your abdomen tighten, as if it were being squeezed. Hold that position for 10 seconds, 15 if you can, then release. Repeat this for ten repetitions.

Scissor kicks.

Lay flat on the floor with your legs out straight. Put your hands by your backside, or under if you prefer. Inhale slowly, and raise one leg as high as is comfortable, but not so high it is at 90 degrees to the floor. As you lower it, slowly raise the other leg. Continue this at least 10 - 15 times, and try and do three sets. If you can't at first, don't worry just build up to it.

Am I too old to exercise?

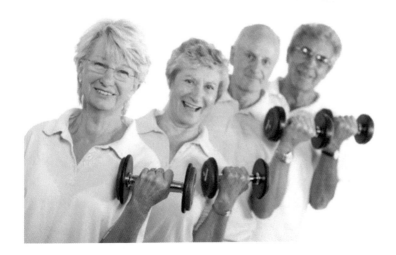

The short answer to this is no, you are never too old to start, or keep going for that matter. Age in and of itself is not a barrier to health and fitness. I once had a Sensei, a martial arts teacher, who was in her mid 70s before she retired from training (to go travelling, no less), and even right up to the end she could run rings around us much younger, much larger men when we were in our prime! Trust me, nothing keeps your ego in check as a young, 6"2, muscular man on his way to earning a black belt as much as being effortlessly put on your backside by a tiny woman in her 70s!

The truth is people in general are living a lot longer than they used to. People hitting their 100th birthday is much more common now and much less of a rare celebration. In some cases medicine is extending lives far beyond what they should be doing, and I know, you may think that sounds strange coming from a nurse. However, the sheer amount of people making poor lifestyle choices throughout their lives has led to the quality of those extended lives in many cases being extremely poor indeed. Chronic degenerative diseases, poor health and a complete lack of quality of life is a reality for many people in the last years, sometimes even decades of their lives. I see daily many examples of elderly people being completely bed bound with no real mobility at all, being unable to breathe without oxygen from years of smoking, having their independence taken away from them due to a stroke or any number of other conditions that have a profound effect on their ability to enjoy life. Having seen it first hand in many of my patients, I do not mind admitting that the idea of having no health or quality of life at all in my later years scares me, and the idea of my loved ones having no quality of life scares me even more

I see a few patients from middle age upwards, often a fair bit later in life, who get shocked into wanting to adopt a healthy lifestyle through a specific injury or serious health scare. Whilst it is good that they are considering it at all, with many it has already become an issue of damage control rather than prevention. Ideally you want to start living a healthy lifestyle long before that. If you don't, well all is not lost.

You can still limit any damage you have done to your body and manage any condition you have developed through prolonged poor lifestyle choices. You can always improve your quality of life through making the right lifestyle choices at any age, but I know I wouldn't want to run that quality of life gauntlet.

The ideal of course, is to live a healthy lifestyle from as early an age as possible, so that you can continue to enjoy your health, vitality and quality of life for as long as you can. But this in reality doesn't always happen. The good news is however is that it is never too late to start. The human body is a wonderful machine that has remarkable healing qualities if you give it the right tools and environment in which to do so. By improving your lifestyle choices, eating a healthy diet and getting some exercise, you can still benefit from improvements to your strength, fitness and general health.

There are a whole myriad of diseases and conditions that are associated with age. The age related risk of coronary heart disease, hypertension (high blood pressure), diabetes mellitus, through to osteoporosis (brittle bones), sarcopenia (muscle wastage) and arthritis, for just a few examples, should be taken into account when undertaking any type of exercise program, but that does not mean that they should be a barrier to it. Clinical research has shown repeatedly that all of these conditions can become much less symptomatic with exercise, or even make you less likely to suffer from them at all! On top of that, you will see and feel benefits in strength, fitness and flexibility, all things that naturally deteriorate with age, so what is stopping you?

How much training should I do as I get older?

This is a very simple question, with a very easy answer. The basic 2 and a half hours each week of moderate cardiovascular exercise, plus strength training on all major muscle groups twice a week that is recommended for adults over 18 is still applicable right up until your 64th Birthday! Of course if you can and want to do more than that then that is absolutely great, I won't discourage you! The more you do the better. After your 64th birthday then it is basically a case of trying to keep it up and doing as much as you can without overdoing it. Just go at your own pace and enjoy it. You yourself will know what your own limits are.

So what training should I do?

Of course there are some things to consider if you start training when you are relatively old, or you continue training into old age. Your training routine will not be the same as someone 30 or 40 years your junior, that much should be pretty obvious. Your body will obviously not be able to perform the same way it did 30, 40 or even 50 years ago. The aches, pains and general unfitness you build up as you get older and older will place more and more barriers in your way, and the accumulative effects of long term health conditions such as heart, lung or kidney disease, arthritis and osteoporosis will take their toll. This does not mean that you should use any of this as an excuse not to start exercising, just that you should modify your training to take any limitations into account.

As you get older, functional fitness is a term that you should become familiar with. This basically means you are not training toward a specific fitness goal such as running a marathon, or training to get to a high level of fitness, but are instead training to ensure that your body can continue to perform the everyday tasks it always has done. This involves doing regular dynamic and static stretches and movement with or without light weights that involve a lot of bending, twisting and stretching. This ensures that your joints maintain their full range of movement (or get it back, if you have started to lose it), and you can continue to live your life and perform your normal activities of daily living. This is a basis of what you should be doing, and if you want or are able to do more and get fitter, then great.

Strength and cardiovascular training are still just as important now as they are at any age, and the exercises outlined in the above chapters are still absolutely fine to do. Don't expect to be running marathons or entering bodybuilding competitions straight away if you have never done much training before, (although there is nothing wrong with having these as goals to aim for) but you can still utilise the full range of cardio, strength and flexibility exercises to become fitter, stronger and healthier. As you get older however, you simply need to modify the ratio, intensity and type of training you do slightly.

Low impact training.

Low impact training is exactly what it sounds like. It consists of a range of exercises that you can do without putting your joints through too much pressure or impact. Regardless of your age, high impact exercises such as running or sports such as Rugby can have a detrimental effect on your joints. All those years spent pounding the pavement or the treadmill can affect your knees if you are not careful, especially if they are carrying a lot of weight. That is why it is recommended to have a variety of training styles in your routine. As you get older, this issue is compounded with issues such as osteoporosis (brittle bones) and arthritis.

Cardiovascular exercise is still vitally important to keep you fit and healthy as you get older. Now I want to make it absolutely clear that there is nothing wrong with high impact exercises such as running, jogging and so on, but should be used increasingly in moderation or in conjunction with low impact exercises as you get older. Low impact workouts are ideal in later years, especially if you suffer from joint and mobility problems as they put much less strain and pressure on your joints whilst giving you a cardiovascular workout. Water workouts such as swimming and aqua aerobics are ideal and are often lauded as one of the best all round workouts as they give you a great cardio workout, as well as the added benefit of forcing you to use your muscles against resistance rather than using heavy weights. This makes your muscles and joints work with very little risk of injury and often alleviate the aches and pains associated with arthritis or osteoporosis.

If you run or jog a lot, either outside or on the treadmill, then that is absolutely great, but try and do more workouts using other cardio equipment too. The cross trainer or the rowing machine for example will still get your heart rate going and give you a cardio workout, whilst giving your knee joints a bit of a rest from the pounding they get when you run.

Strength training is absolutely important too, especially as you get older and have to combat sarcopenia (muscle wastage). If you are used to strength training or weights training, then there is absolutely no reason why you cannot carry on into your elder years too as long as you take into account specific advice to train safely and effectively. There are many examples of middle aged or elderly body builders for example who have continued their training. Many people do not need to go to this extreme however, and if you find that you naturally cannot lift as much weight as you could twenty years ago or your joints can't handle the pressure of a heavy barbell press, then that is fine, you just have to adjust your training to take your age into account. It is perhaps more important to train for endurance, flexibility and simple range of movement as you get older as opposed to pure strength and power, so use lighter weights instead but perform a lot more reps and sets to train your slow twitch muscle fibres or simply use them to ensure that you can maintain a full range of movement with all your joints and limbs.

Many people substitute weights for resistance training as they get older, especially if they have not had a significant background in using weights. This involves the use of rubber bands of different tensile strength. The exercises performed are very similar to their weighted counterparts, such as the bicep curl for example, but will have you pulling on a large rubber band attached to an apparatus or your feet instead of lifting a weight. This type of training is fantastic for promoting range of movement and toning your muscles without adding too much strain on your joints.

Try to incorporate much more flexibility training and stretching into any routine, especially if it has never factored much in your life before, as flexibility becomes a serious issue in your later years if you let it. Tai Chi, Pilates and Yoga are perfect for this, as this will help you to maintain good posture, flexibility and mobility as well as improving your joint's range of movement. They are often considered 'gentle' exercises that are perfect for the elderly, and whilst it is true that they are a great exercise form for any age group, they do have qualities that are ideal for training in your later years.

There are so many ways to tailor any exercise to your age and individual requirements, but always remember to seek advice from both health and fitness professionals before you even start doing anything, as they can take your own specific medical and fitness history into account when giving you advice on what to do.

The most important thing to remember is that by doing exercise and living a healthy lifestyle, you will quite simply live better as well as live longer. It is about much, much more than simply increasing the amount of years you have, it is about staying active and healthy throughout those years too. With exercise and a healthy lifestyle you will have a quality of life much longer than you would do otherwise, and you will be able to enjoy life for a lot longer as a result.

Part 4 - So what now?

I hope by now that you have read the advice contained in this book and have not only seen how relatively simple it is to eat a healthy diet, incorporate a minimum level of exercise into your daily routine and look after your health and wellbeing, but have also been inspired to make that commitment toward living a healthy lifestyle over the long term.

Feeling fitter, faster, stronger, healthier!

If you have followed the advice in this book and you have really made an effort to eat a healthier diet and incorporate exercise into your life, then after just a short month, you should already start to feel a lot better about yourself. It may only be the small things you notice at first, being able to breathe normally after climbing the stairs, being able to play with the kids without falling down in a tearful, wheezing heap, feeling like you have more energy or a general feeling of wellbeing, it doesn't matter. The point is you should be feeling much better in just a short period of time!

Making the right choices.

I hope that in some way, this book has made you take a little bit of an honest look at your own lifestyle choices, without the benefit of all the rose tinted glasses, little white lies and outright excuses that we all make at some point or another, and has in some way inspired you to make the right choices for the future. Eating healthily, getting some exercise and living a healthier lifestyle. It doesn't matter how you do it as long as you do. Whether you choose to join a gym or exercising at home, learning how to cook fresh meals from scratch or starting slow by just cutting down on the really unhealthy stuff at first. The point is, you are making the right choices that will really benefit you and your quality of life. Now I know once you have made the decision to live a healthier lifestyle, there are still a few important decisions to consider, and there is no right and wrong answer here. What is right for one person may not be right for another. What the next section aims to do is to give you a few facts and a few things to consider to make those decisions just a little bit easier.

Choosing a gym.

If you do decide that using a gym is the right course of action for you, then it is important that you choose the right one. There are as many different gyms as there are differing training needs, so don't just pick the first one you come across because it has a fancy brand name and your mum's friend's second cousin twice removed goes there, that is almost certainly a route to giving up going very quickly and then sitting at home crying when your monthly direct debits come in.

When choosing a gym, it really does pay to shop around. Have a look at as many different ones in your area as you can. Ask to be shown around and see if you like it. Ask yourself does it have the right equipment that you would want to use or would fit in with your training goals. There is no point in picking a gym with no free weights area if you want to build muscle for example. Does it have a wide range of classes that you think you might enjoy going to or specifically want to train in? Does it have fully qualified and experienced staff who can help you achieve your goals, or does it seem completely bereft of trainers as you walk around? Don't be afraid of asking these questions either, the trainers and instructors are there to help you but all of them will have their own specific areas of expertise, so if you want help or guidance in a particular area, it can really help to get someone who is an expert who can help you meet your individual fitness goals. Ask how busy the gym gets and if there are quiet times too, because if you like training alone there is absolutely nothing worse than having to wait for equipment to become available. Especially if there are groups of people using the place as a social club and chatting instead of training. All these things and more make such a difference when choosing the right gym, believe me, and choosing the right gym can make all the difference in keeping your motivation up and training well.

Training at home.

If you decide for whatever reason that a gym just isn't for you then there is absolutely nothing wrong with that. Training at home or even outside can be just as good when done right. Again, the key is to make the right choices to make it a valid option.

Space is vital, so ask yourself honestly do you really have enough space to devote to training at home. A devoted room is ideal, but the living room is okay too as long as you can ensure you can push the furniture out of the way. There is nothing worse than cracking your ankle on the coffee table when the jumping round to the fitness DVD gets out of hand, apart from maybe seeing that the old couple walking the dog past your living room window just saw the whole thing.

Choosing the right equipment is really important too. There are a huge variety of ways to train at home now, from buying very basic equipment such as stability balls through to entire home gyms. The choice of equipment is mind boggling. Starting simply and cheaply is the key. The last thing you want is to buy an expensive treadmill only to use it as nothing more than an expensive clothes rack in the spare bedroom, and be honest, how many of you know someone who has done that? Simple, basic equipment that you can easily store away, and can easily use on your own without too much guidance or training. Cheap dumbbells, stability balls, or even resistance bands are perfect for this scenario.

Perhaps the most important thing when training at home is motivation. No you can't just finish watching that episode of Midsummer. No you can't just give yourself another twenty minutes. Get away from the fridge and put that bundle of washing down! Stop procrastinating! If you are home for long enough that you want to train there, then set aside a specific time to do so and stick to it, keep exercising for the full length of time you designated too, just as you would do if you had actually gone to the gym.

Put that cake down and slowly back away from the fridge!

If you have made all the right choices so far and have made a real effort to exercise and eat healthily, then it would be a shame to spoil all of that by slipping back into your old habits. Remember what you read in previous chapters, there is absolutely nothing at all wrong with giving yourself the occasional chocolate bar or takeaway as a treat, as long as it is a treat. Making the right choices on a day to day basis, putting the effort in to cook a meal the majority of the time instead of taking the easy option will keep you on the right track and stop you going back to your old, unhealthy ways.

The long game.

Changing your lifestyle and following the advice contained in this book will not be easy at first, it will take a little effort on your part and real dedication to transform your life. But if you do, if you follow the advice contained within this book and make those changes, then you will have greatly reduced the chances of suffering some serious long term health conditions caused by poor lifestyle choices and you will be much fitter, much healthier and will look and feel better than you probably have done in a long time.

Remember however that this change must incorporate your whole lifestyle and be over the long term. There are no such thing as quick fix diets. There is no point in grabbing a few pieces of fruit in the weekly shop in an effort to start eating healthy, and then going back to the microwave meals the week after. There is no point in exercising for a couple of weeks in January after you have made your new year's resolutions, if by February you have gone back to your old ways because it is easier. No one will be there to drag you off the couch and kick your backside all the way to the gym, no one will be there to follow you around the supermarket and remove those ready meals as you put them in your trolley. No one will force you to stop smoking or drinking to excess so often. Only you can do all of this. Only you can make the conscious decision to live a healthy lifestyle.

Of course there are a variety of health and fitness professionals and experts who can help, advise and encourage you along the way, but at the end of the day the buck stops with you. You are the only one responsible for your own health.

Hopefully by starting on this path, you will use this book and the advice it contains and incorporate healthier choices into your day to day life. You will see just how quickly the difficulty factor decreases as you become used to the new, healthy lifestyle. Cooking fresh, balanced meals and eating a relatively healthy diet will become second nature to you, you won't think twice about chopping up a load of vegetables and throwing them in a wok for a stir fry and your microwave will start to gather dust as you use it less and less. You will start to wonder how you used to cope without going to the gym a few times a week. In fact, you will eventually reach the point where if you take the occasional week or two off to have a holiday sitting by the pool (we're all entitled to that from time to time), you will find that your body feels horrible, your body will tell you that it isn't being used and isn't running at its best and you will be aching to get back into the gym! Don't believe me? Keep up the exercise over the long term, and you will soon see.

The fact is, once you have reached this point, living a healthy lifestyle will be like second nature to you. You will simply just do it without even thinking. I know it may not seem like that now as you struggle to break old routines and old habits, but it is absolutely true. Put the effort in now, and you will reap the rewards tenfold in the future. The important part right now is remembering that you can do it. It doesn't matter whether you are young or old, male or female, generally healthy or have daily competitions with yourself to find new ways to abuse your body, everyone can make changes to live healthier, be fitter, be better. Everyone can live a healthy lifestyle, you just have to want it.

Printed in Great Britain
by Amazon